I0446941

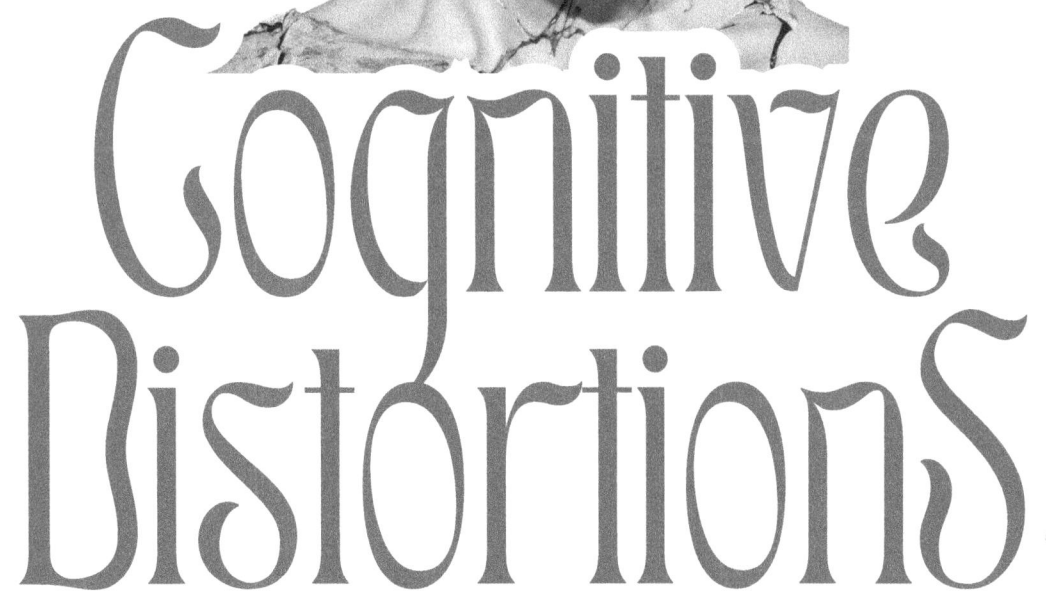

Cognitive Distortions

✳ RECOGNIZE AND CHALLENGE YOUR NEGATIVE THOUGHTS ✳

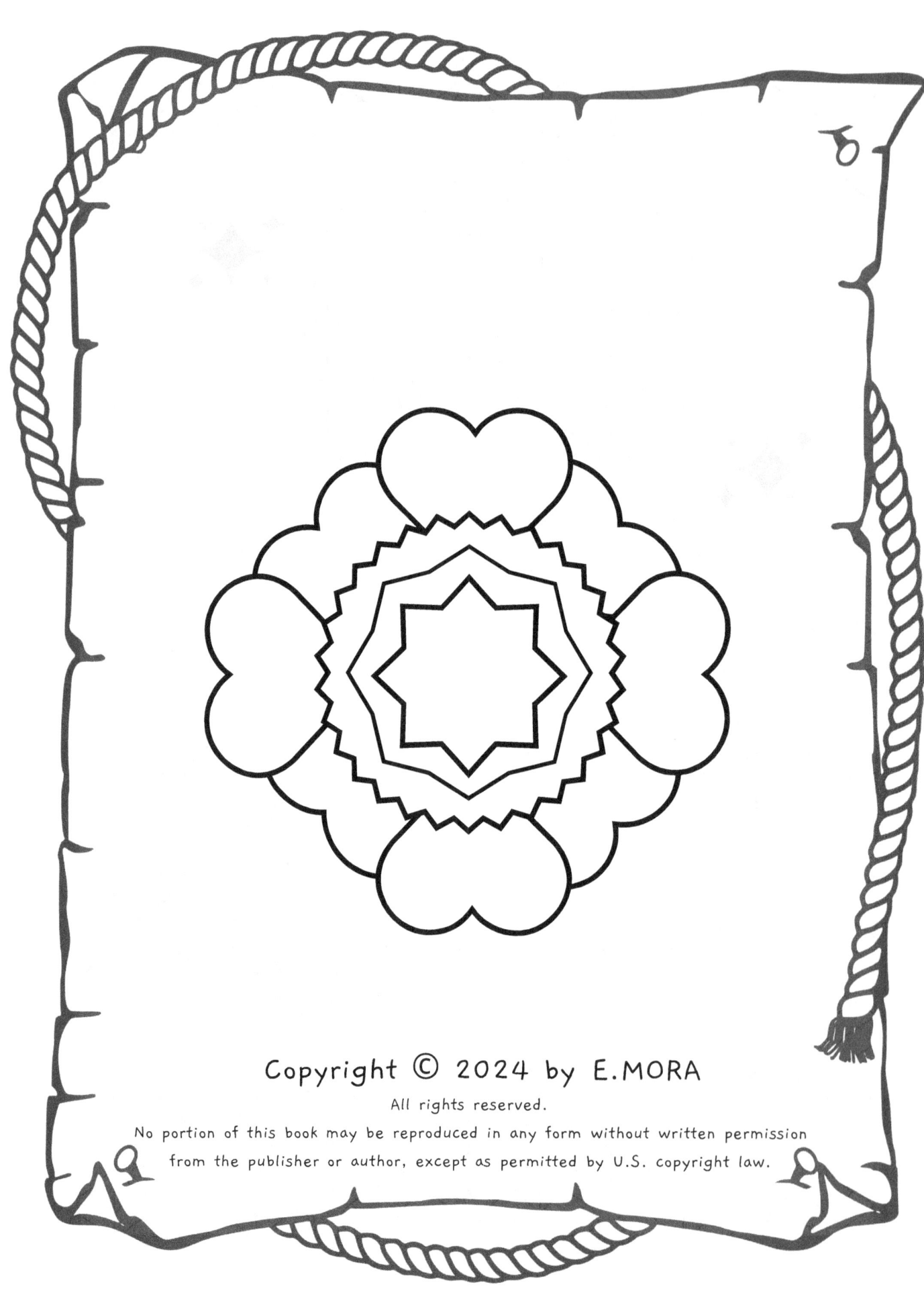

Copyright © 2024 by E.MORA

All rights reserved.

No portion of this book may be reproduced in any form without written permission
from the publisher or author, except as permitted by U.S. copyright law.

All-or-Nothing Thinking

- Distortion: Seeing things in black-and-white categories.
- Challenge: Consider the shades of gray; things are rarely all good or all bad.

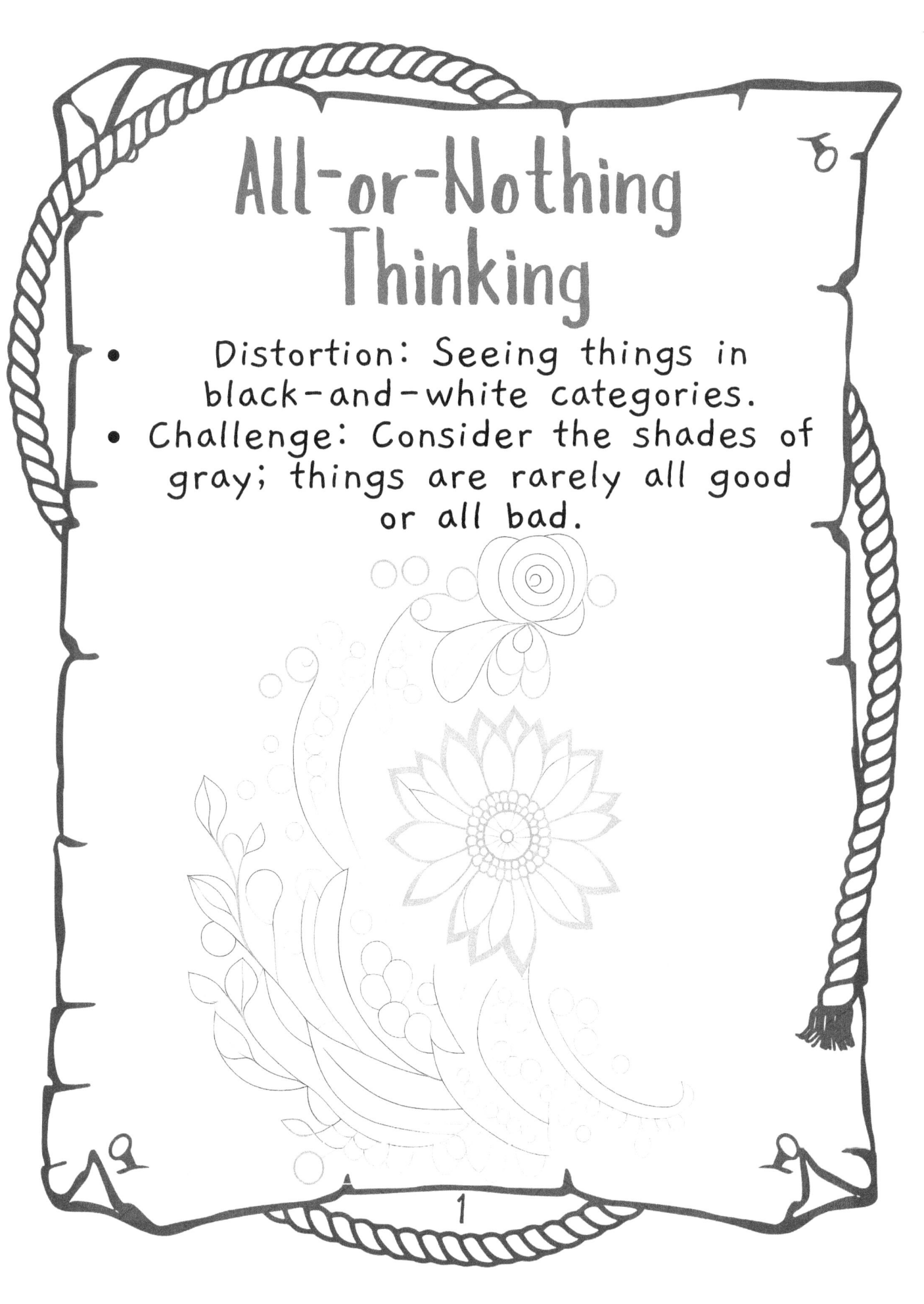

Overgeneralization:

- Distortion: Making broad conclusions based on a single incident.
- Challenge: Look for exceptions to your negative beliefs; not every setback predicts a pattern.

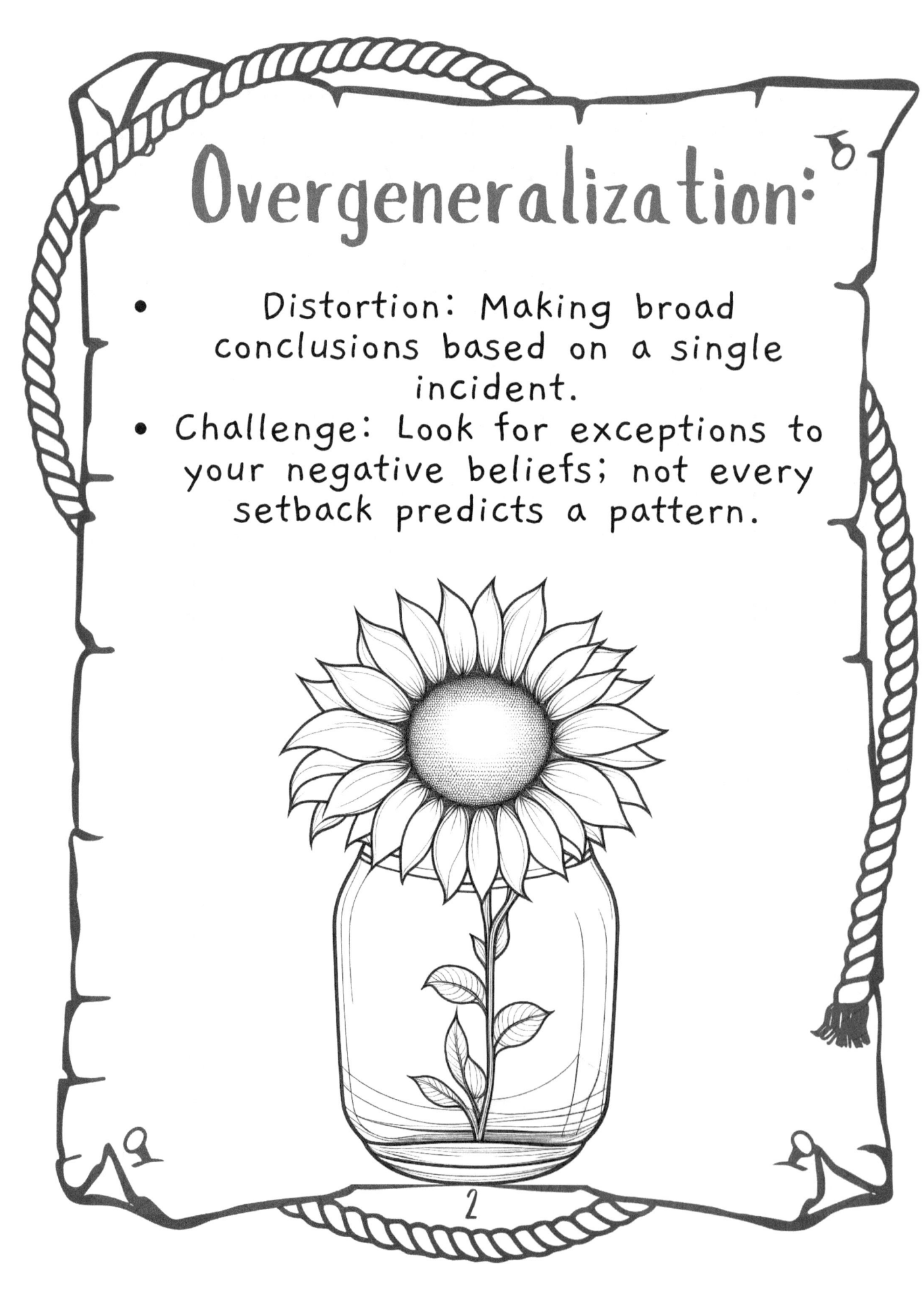

Filtering:

- Distortion: Focusing exclusively on the negative details while ignoring the positive.
- Challenge: Balance your perspective by acknowledging both positive and negative aspects.

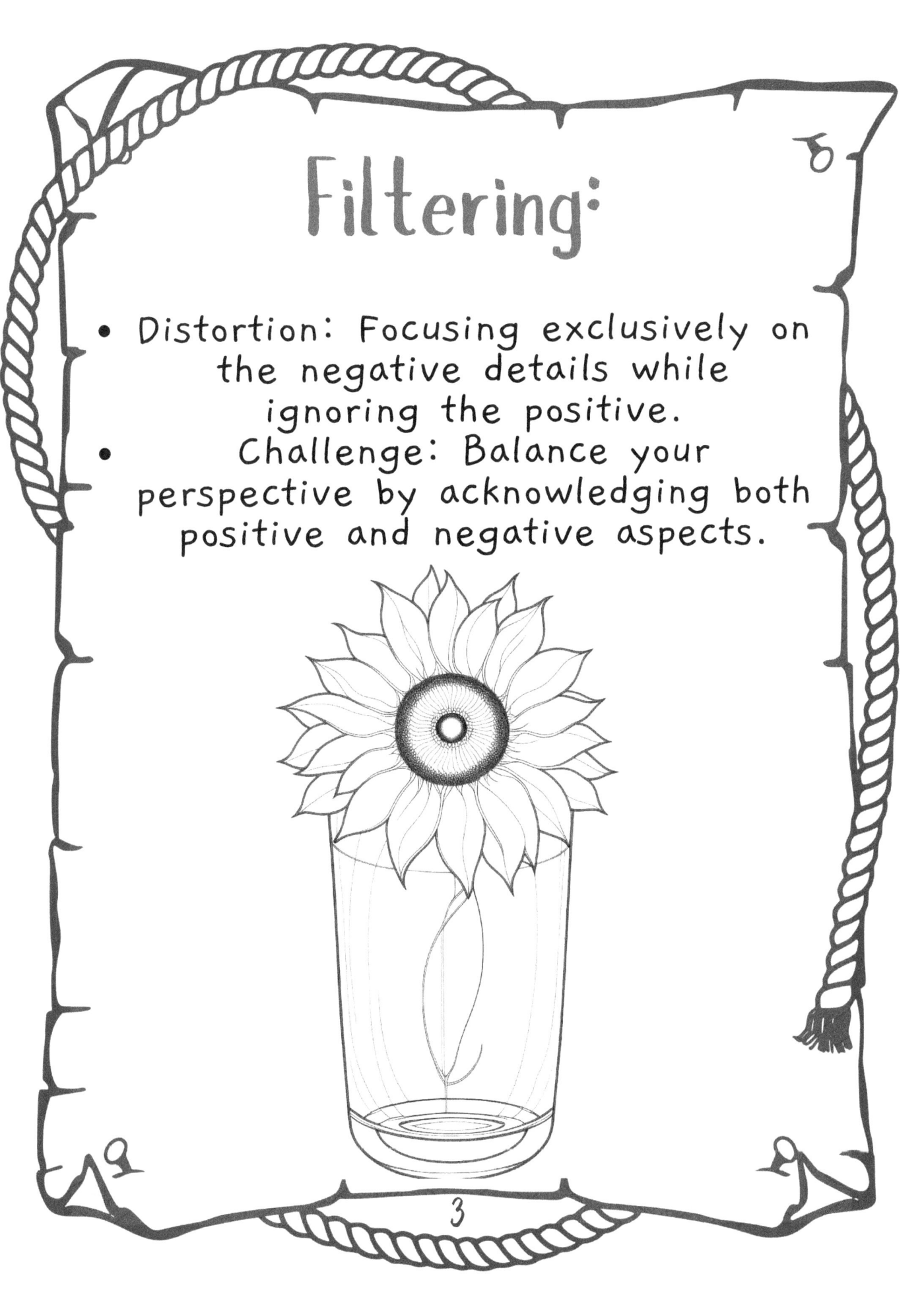

3

Catastrophizing

- Distortion: Expecting the worst-case scenario to happen.
- Challenge: Evaluate the likelihood of your feared outcomes and consider more realistic possibilities.

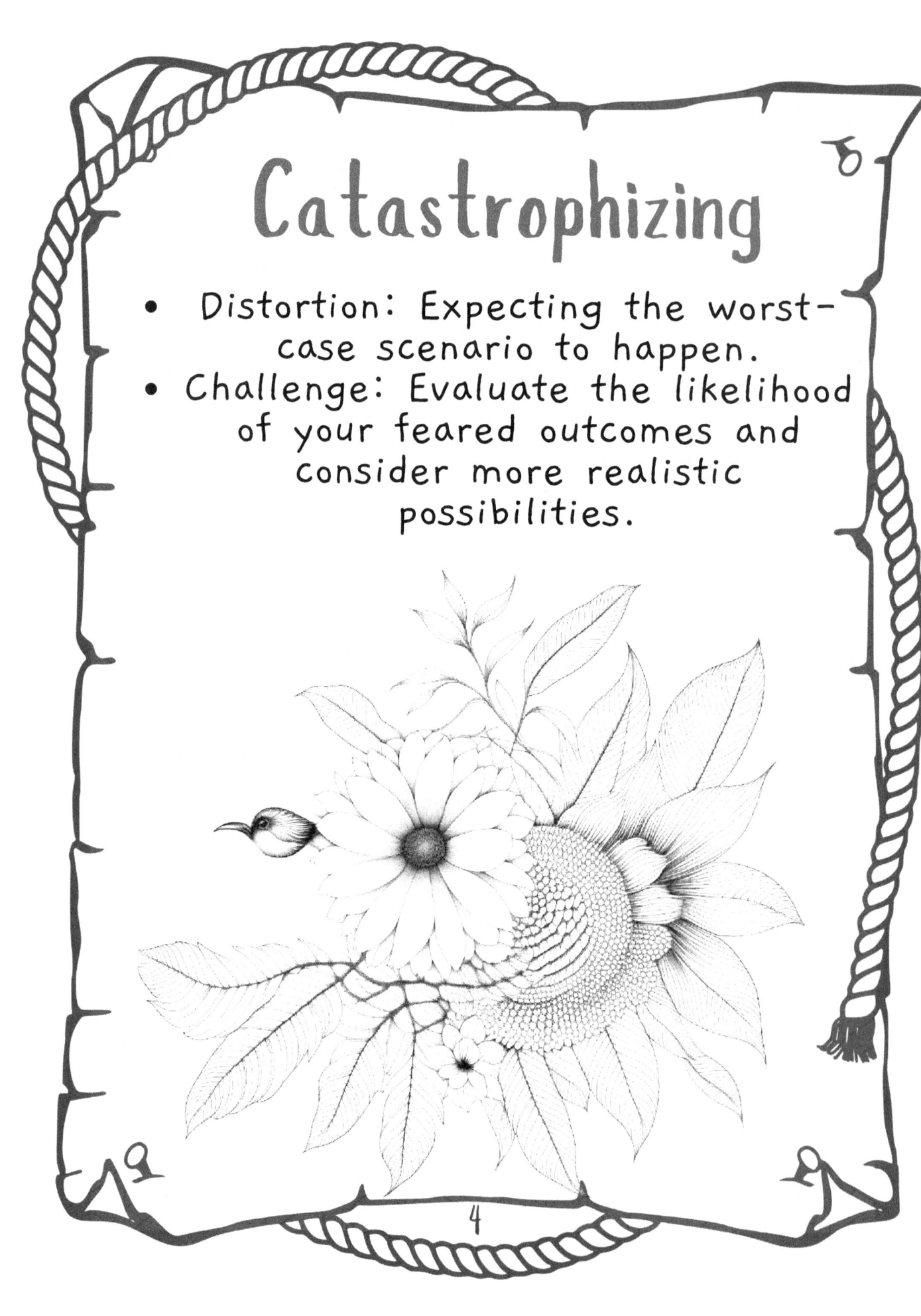

Mind Reading:

- Distortion: Assuming you know what others are thinking.
- Challenge: Seek clarification from others; don't rely on assumptions about their thoughts.

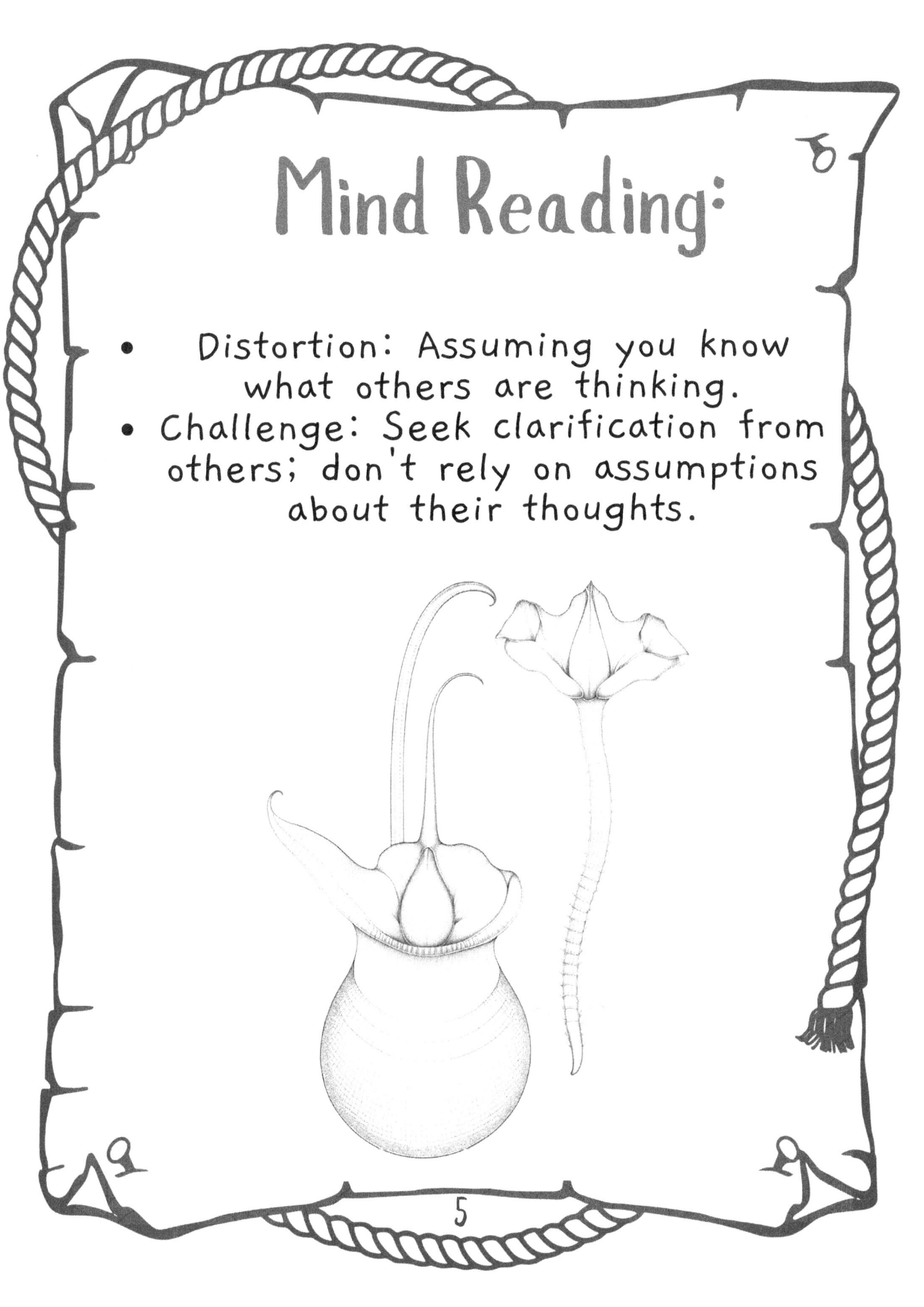

Personalization:

- Distortion: Blaming yourself for external events beyond your control.
- Challenge: Recognize that you are not solely responsible for everything that happens.

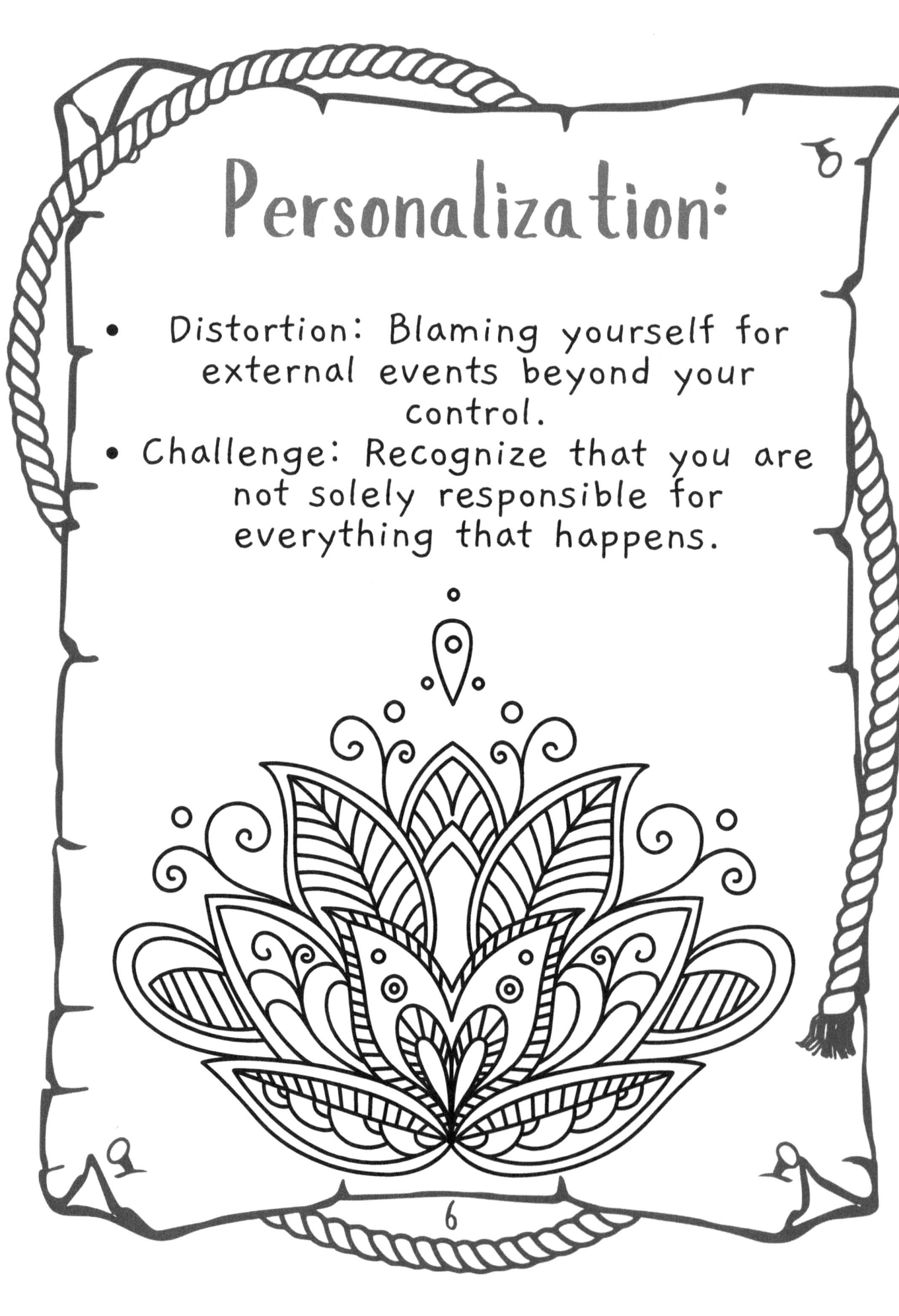

Control Fallacies:

- Distortion: Believing you are helpless in the face of events.
- Challenge: Identify aspects you can control and take positive actions within those limits.

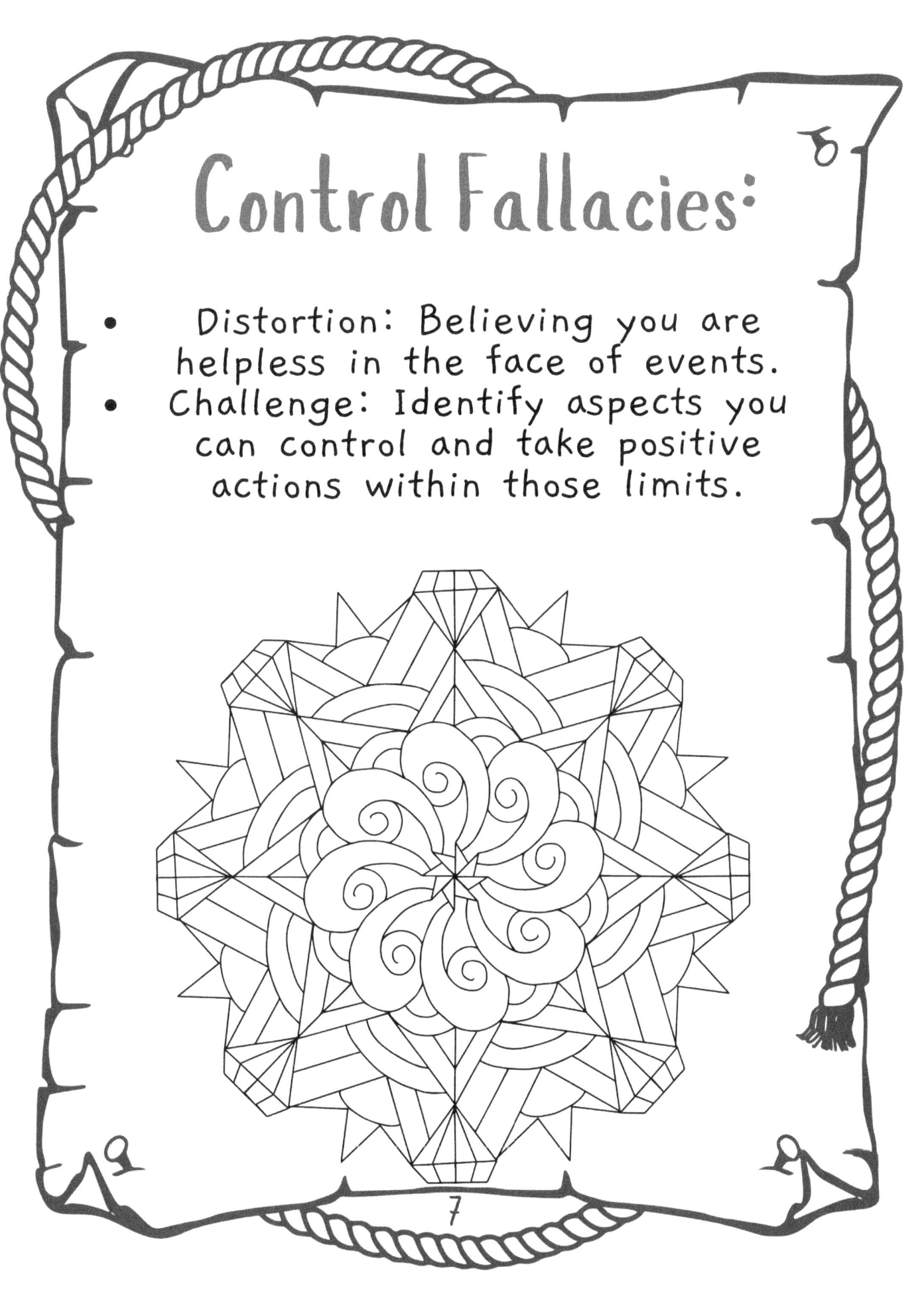

Blaming:

- Distortion: Holding others responsible for your pain.
- Challenge: Focus on what you can do to improve the situation instead of assigning blame.

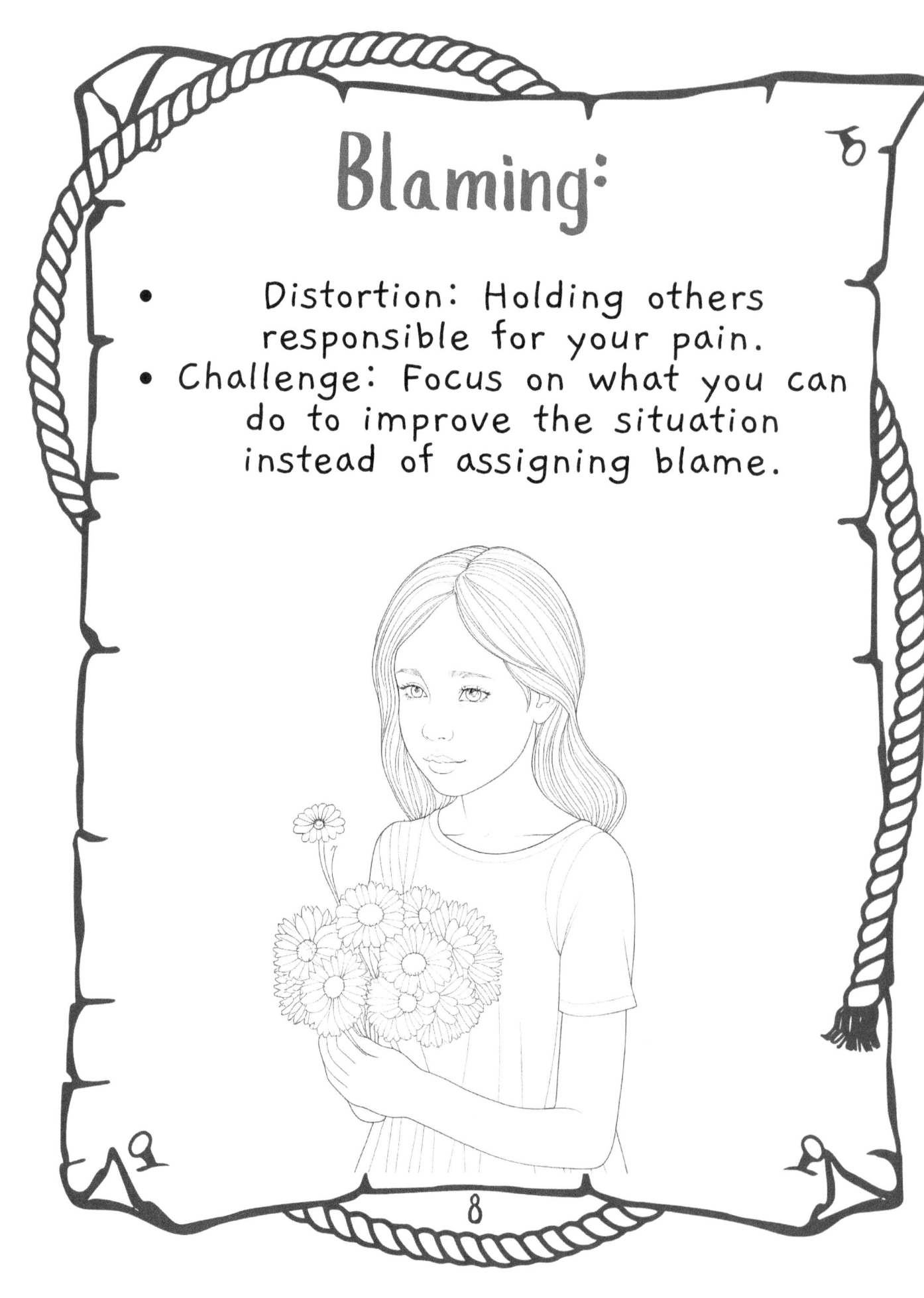

Should Statements:

- Distortion: Having a rigid set of rules about how you and others should behave.
- Challenge: Replace "should" with more flexible language, allowing for realistic expectations.

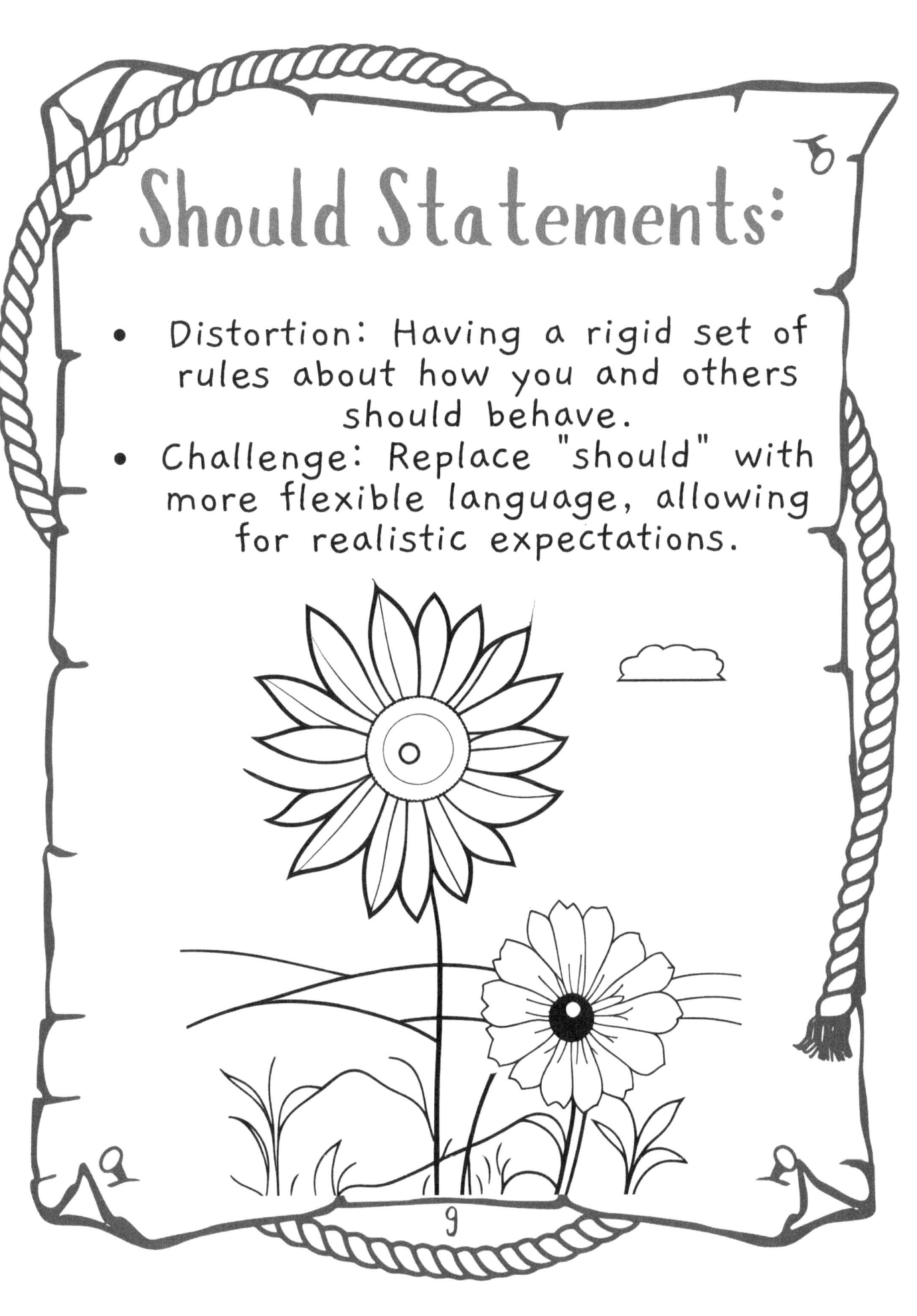

Emotional Reasoning:

- Distortion: Believing that because you feel a certain way, it must be true.
- Challenge: Examine the evidence supporting or contradicting your emotions.

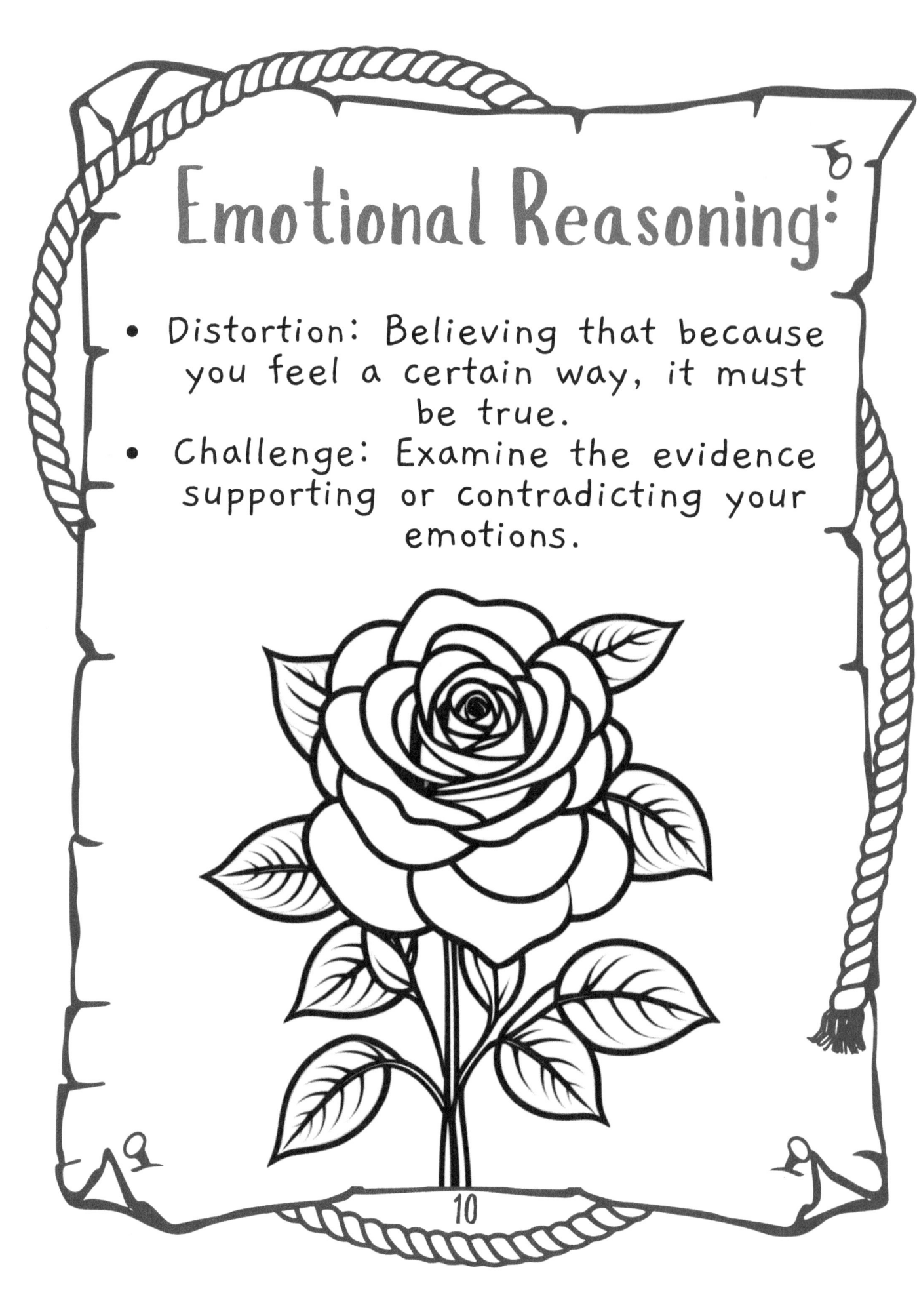

Fallacy of Fairness:

- Distortion: Feeling resentful because you think life should be fair.
- Challenge: Accept that life is not always fair, but you can still make positive changes.

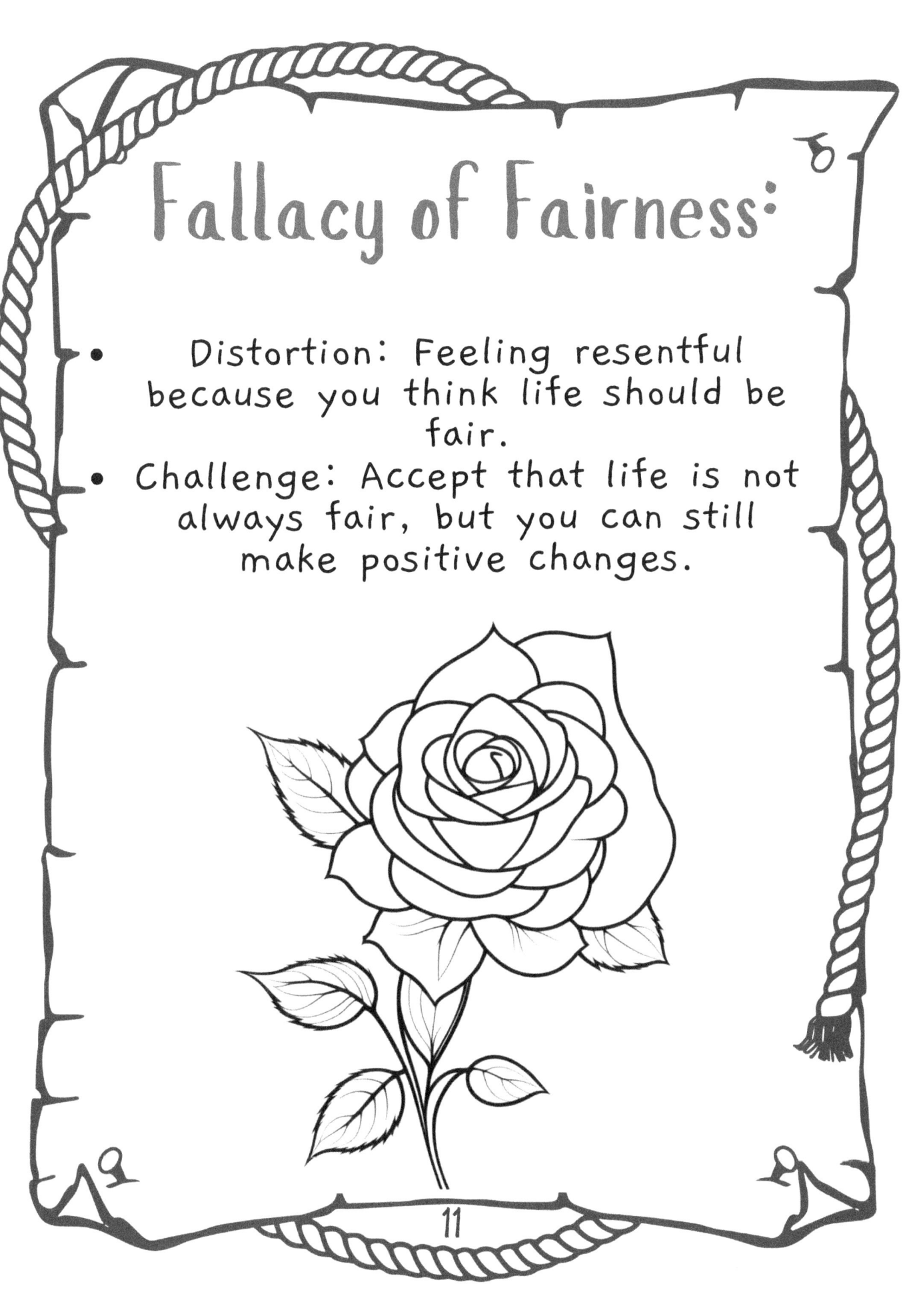

Labeling:

- Distortion: Assigning global, negative labels to yourself or others.
- Challenge: Focus on specific behaviors rather than making sweeping judgments.

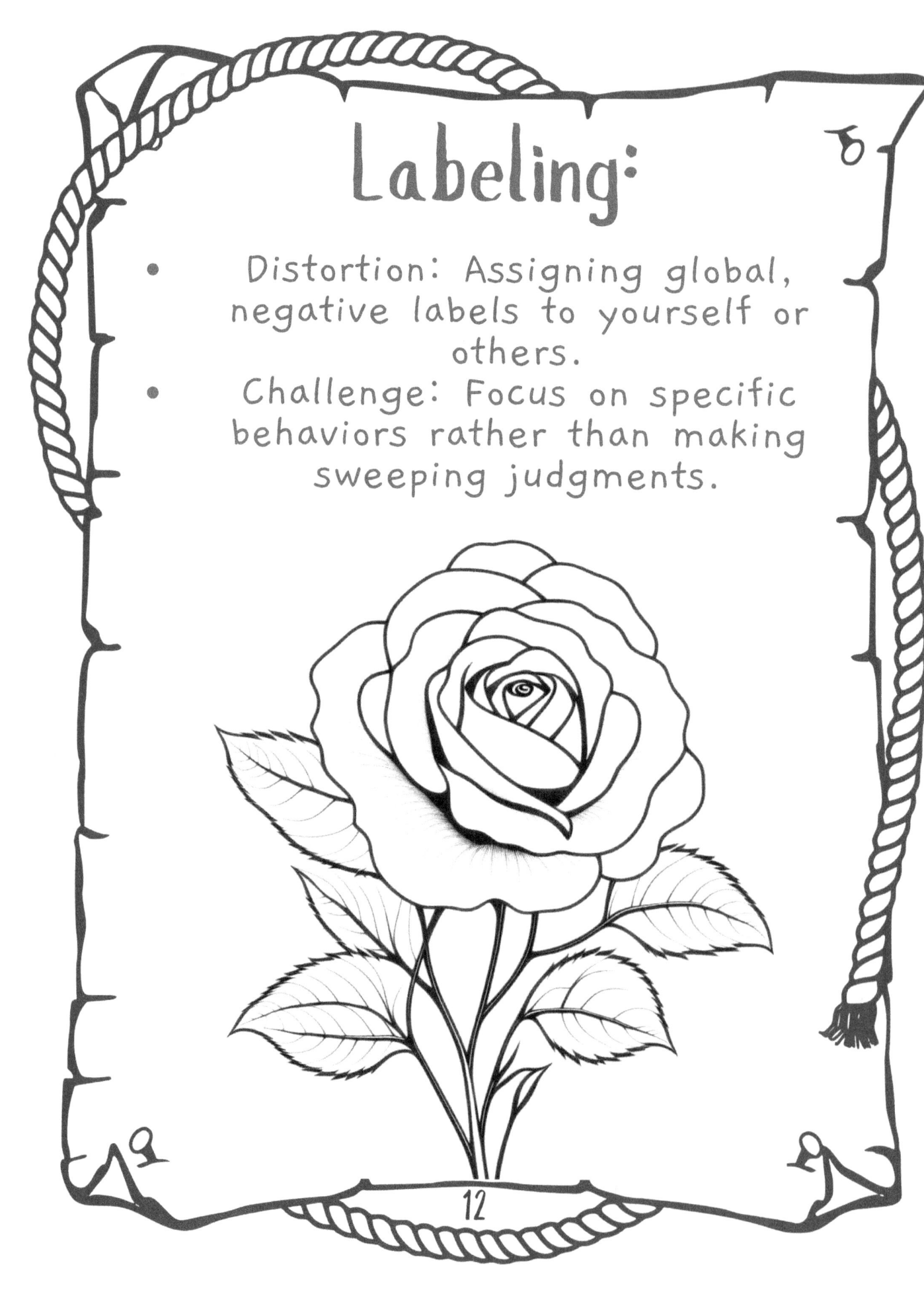

Fortune Telling:

- Distortion: Predicting that things will turn out badly.
- Challenge: Look for evidence that supports or refutes your predictions.

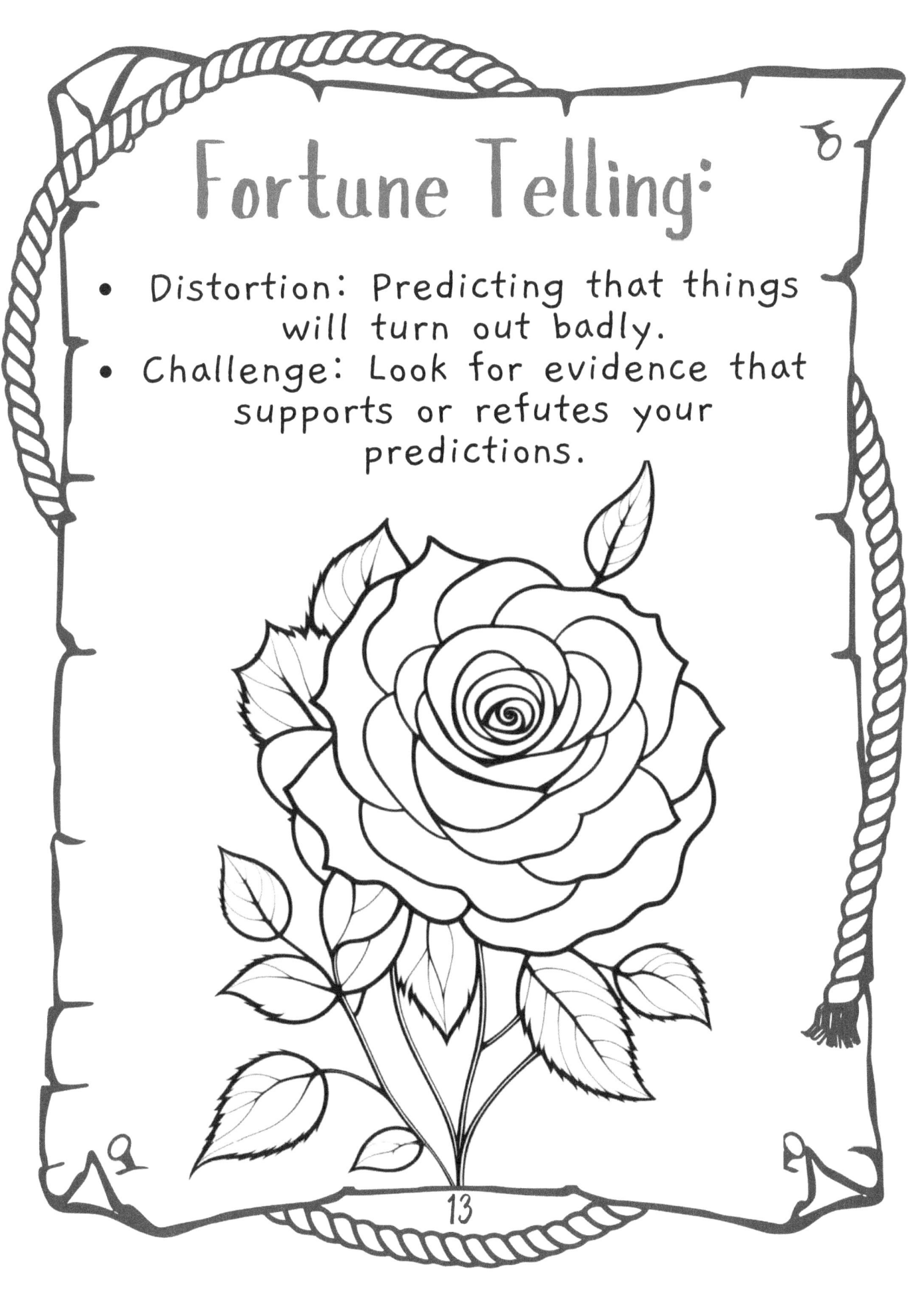

13

Magnification and Minimization:

- Distortion: Exaggerating the importance of negative events or minimizing positive ones.
- Challenge: Balance the significance of events more realistically.

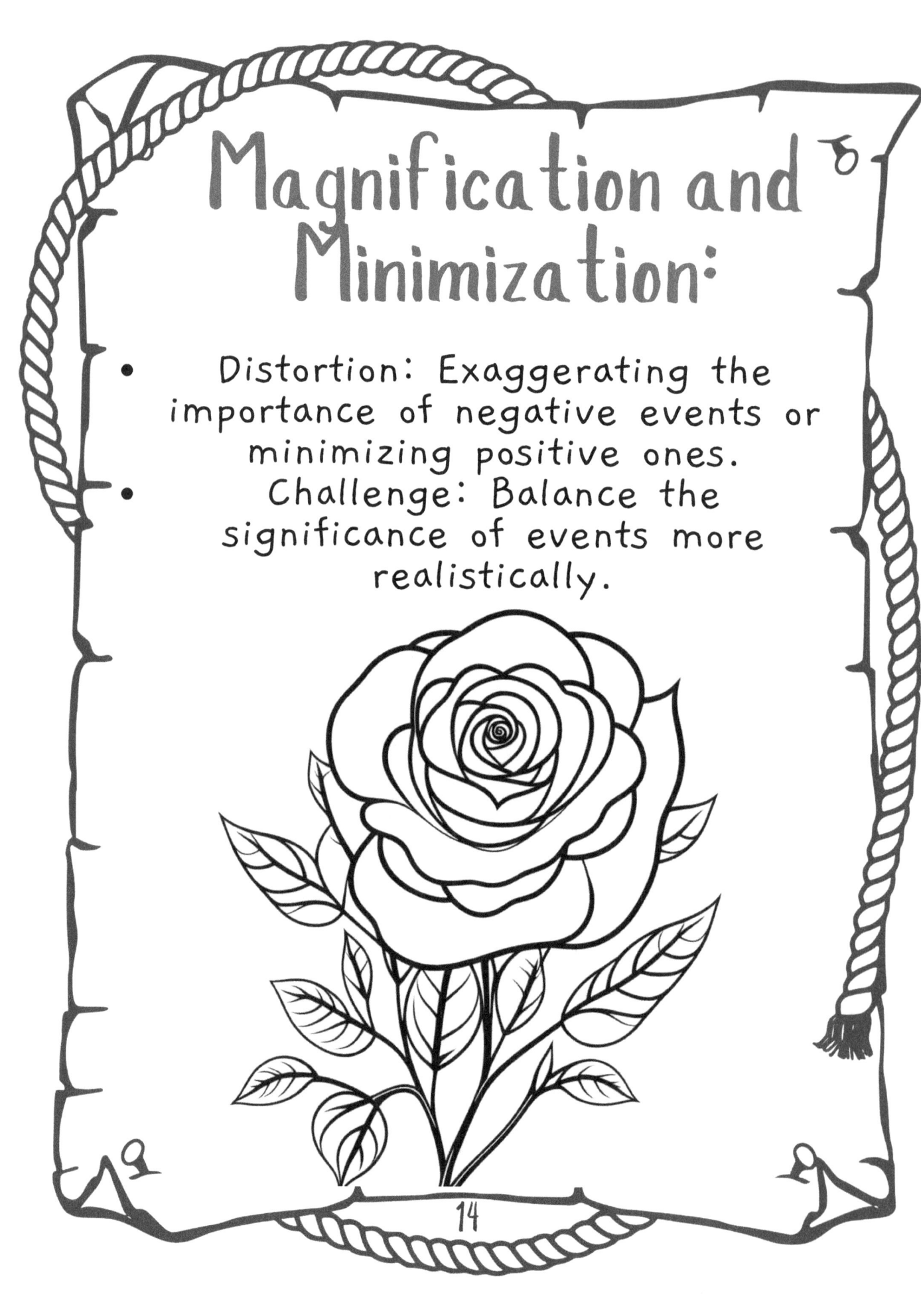

Discounting the Positive:

- Distortion: Insisting that positive experiences "don't count."
- Challenge: Acknowledge and savor positive moments; they are valid and meaningful.

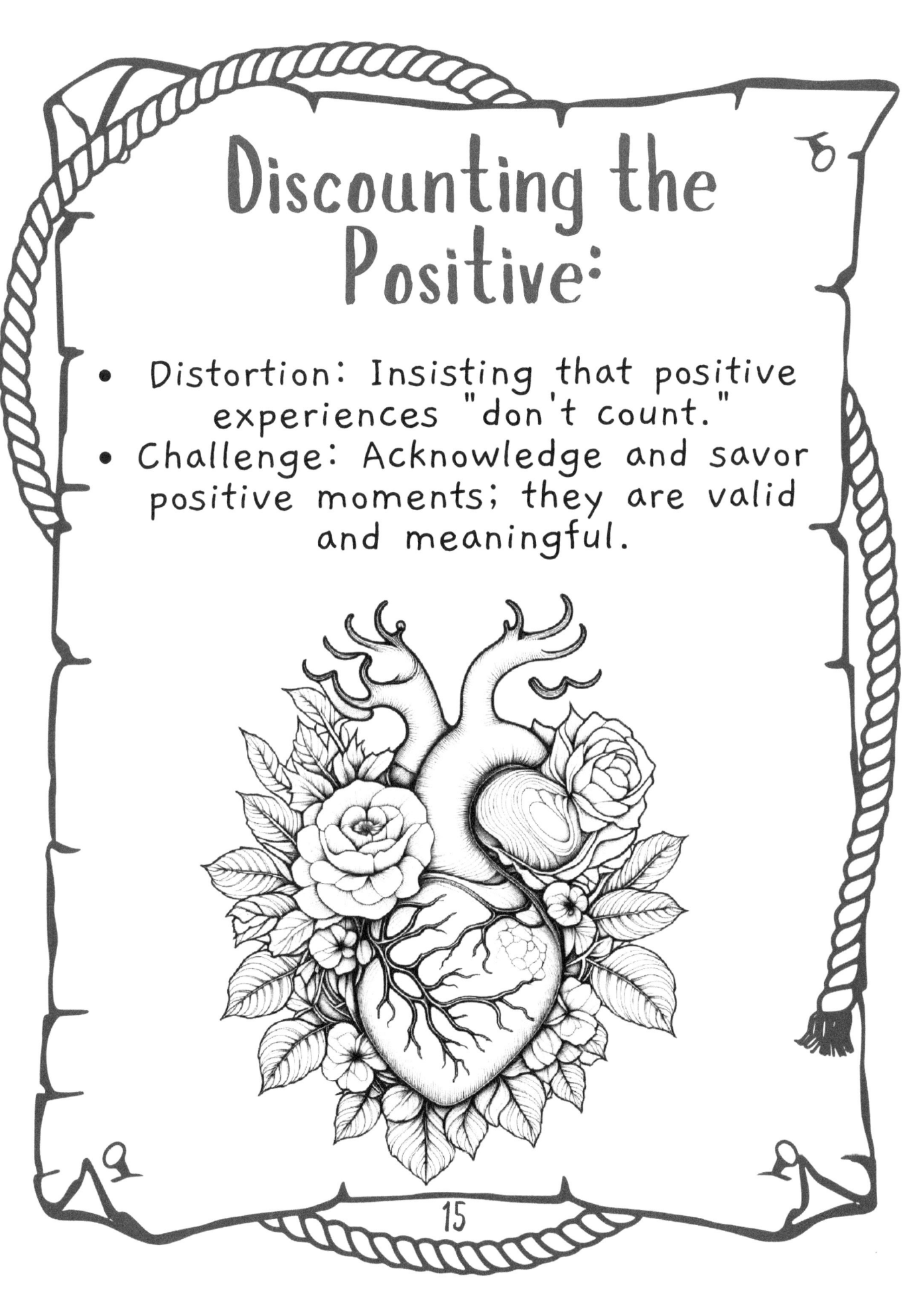

Jumping to Conclusions:

- Distortion: Making negative interpretations without evidence.
- Challenge: Gather more information before reaching conclusions; consider alternative explanations.

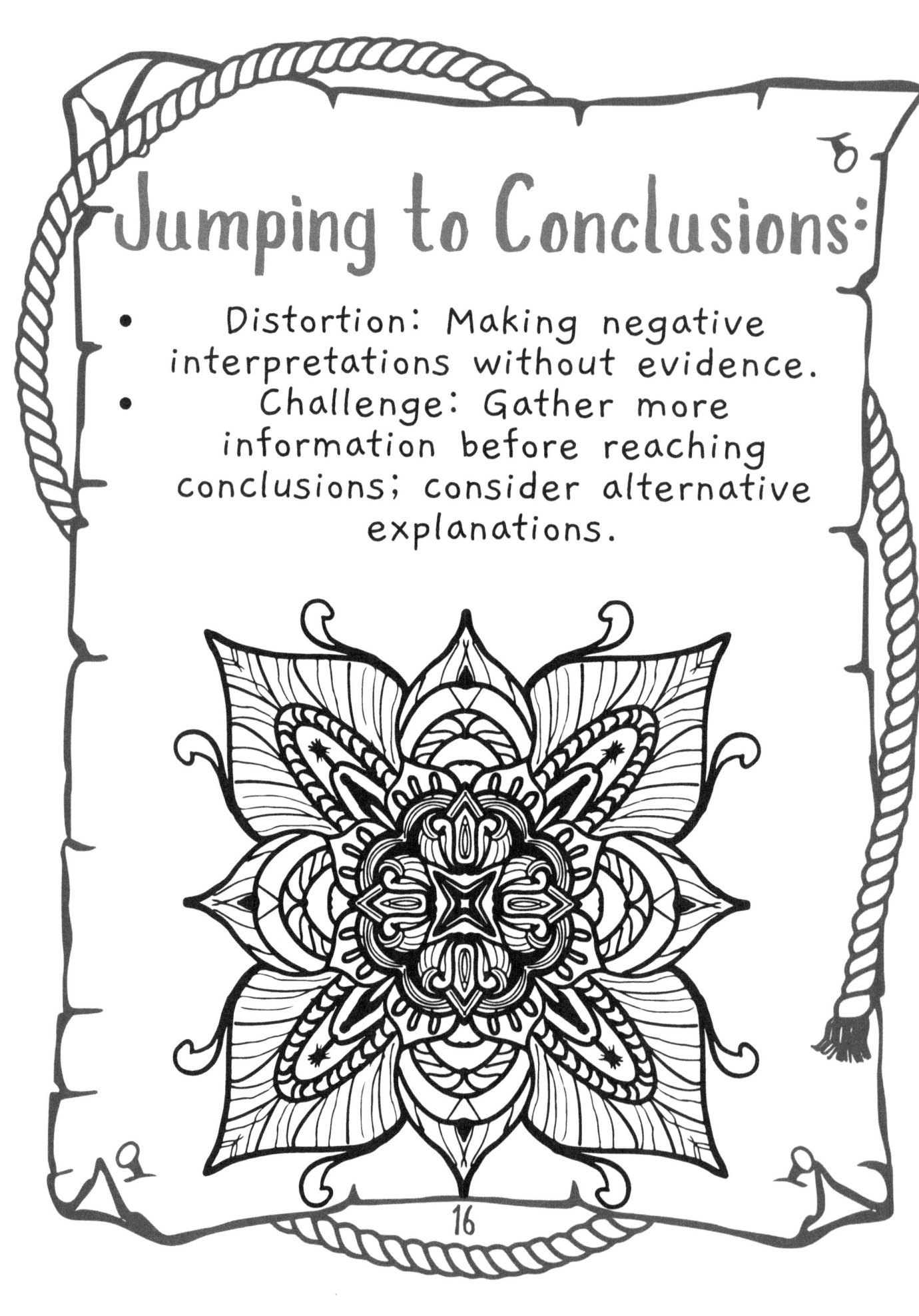

MANDALA
COLORING

Comparisons:

- Distortion: Judging your own worth based on others' achievements.
- Challenge: Focus on your progress and accomplishments rather than comparing yourself to others.

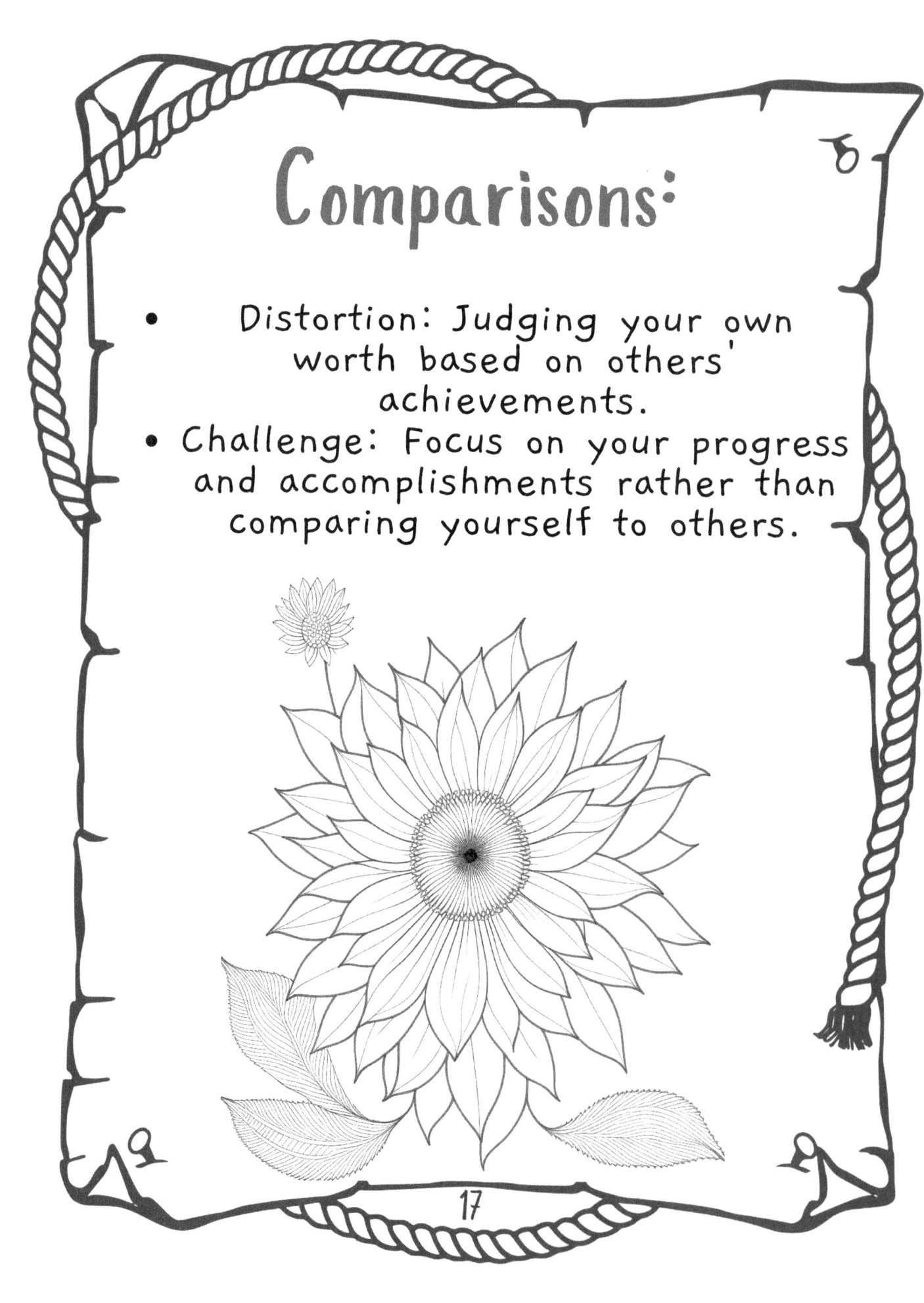

Always Being Right:

- Distortion: Insisting on being right and refusing to admit when you are wrong.
- Challenge: Embrace the idea that learning and growth often come from acknowledging mistakes.

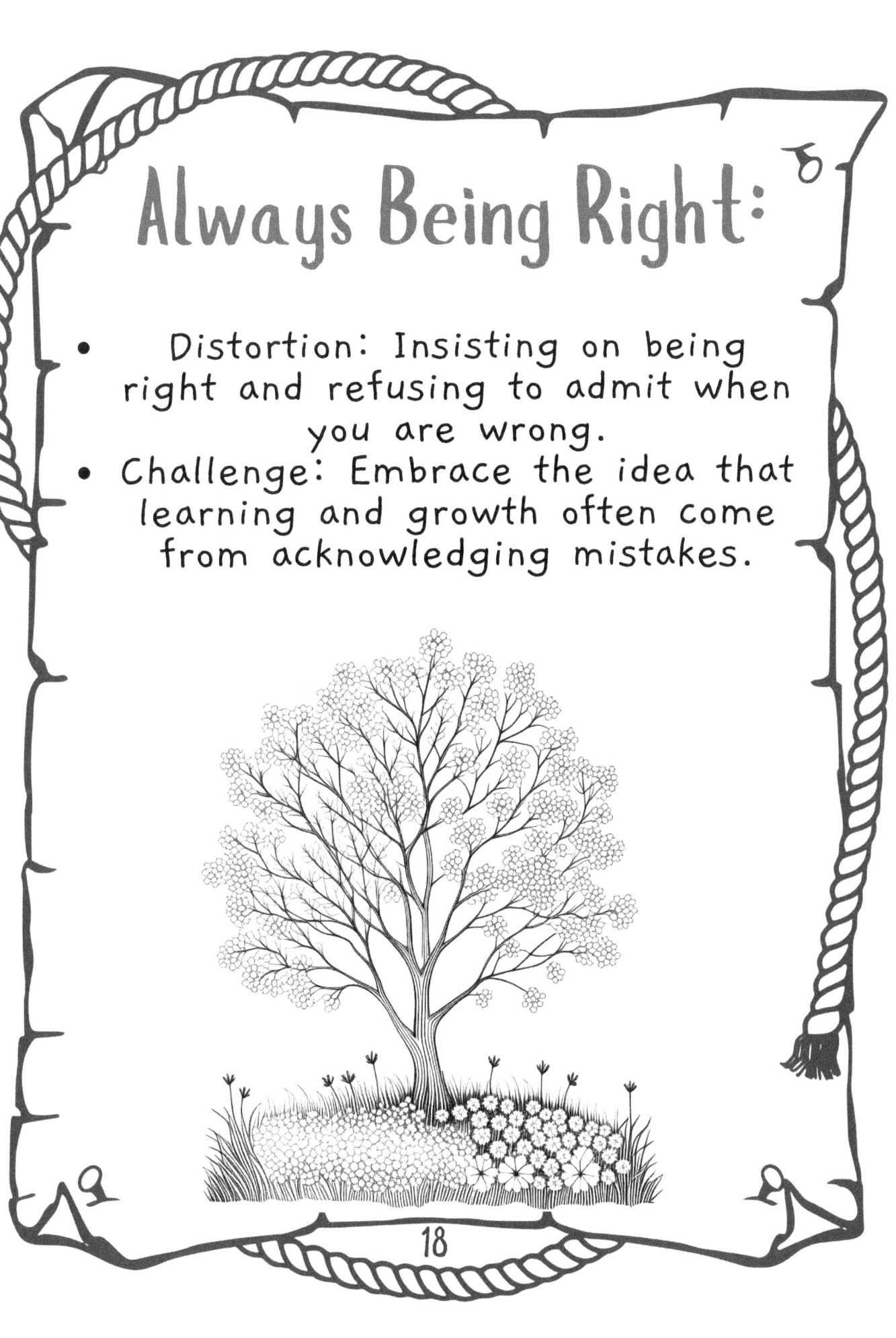

Heaven's Reward Fallacy:

- Distortion: Believing that sacrificing your needs for others will lead to a perfect life.
- Challenge: Balance your priorities and recognize that self-care is essential for overall well-being.

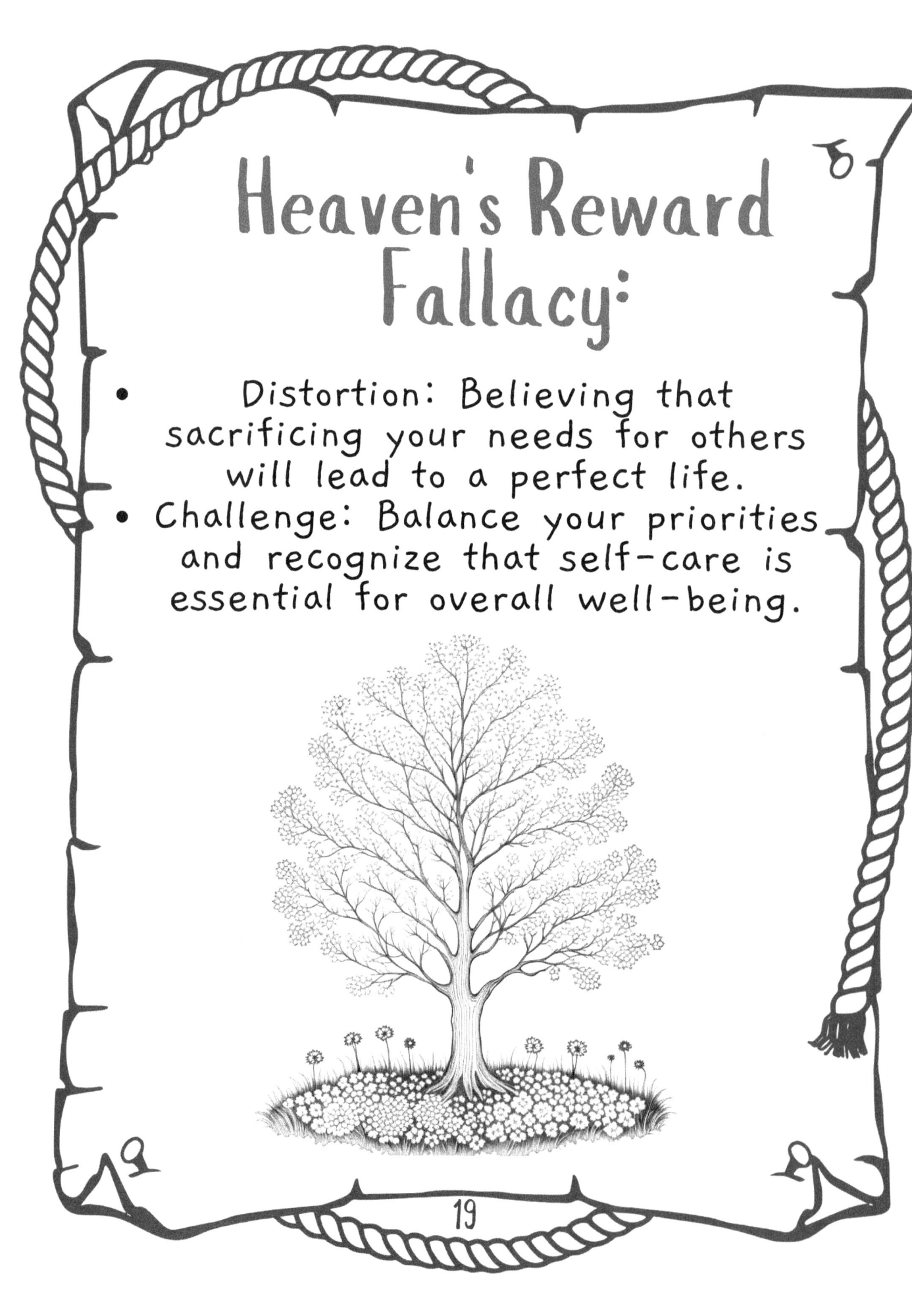

Approval Seeking:

- Distortion: Valuing others' approval over your own feelings.
- Challenge: Prioritize your own values and opinions, seeking internal validation.

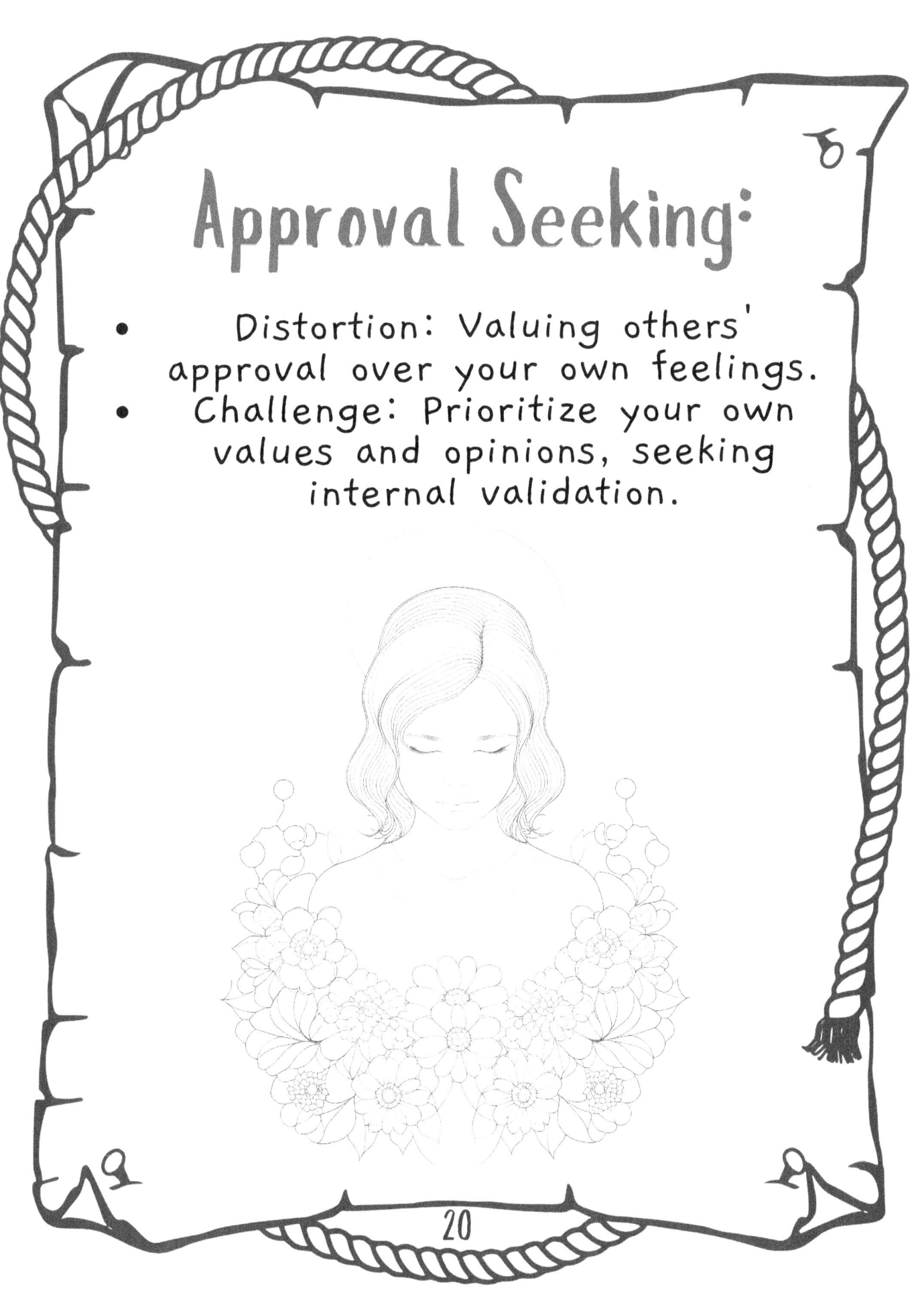

Selective Attention:

- Distortion: Focusing only on certain aspects of a situation, typically the negative ones.
- Challenge: Expand your awareness to include positive elements, providing a more comprehensive view.

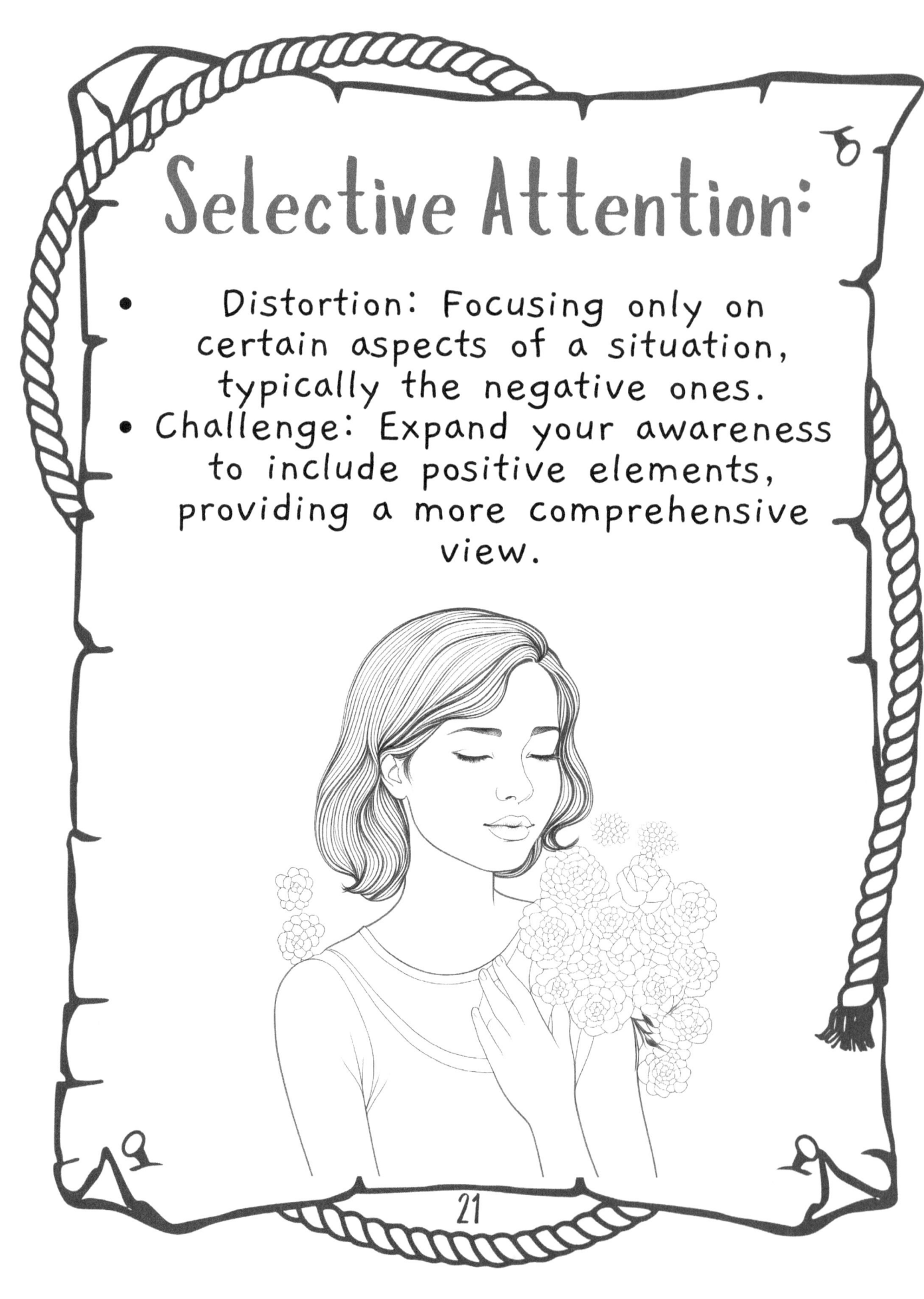

Binary Thinking:

- Distortion: Viewing situations as either/or, without considering middle ground or compromise.
- Challenge: Explore alternative solutions and recognize the diversity of possibilities.

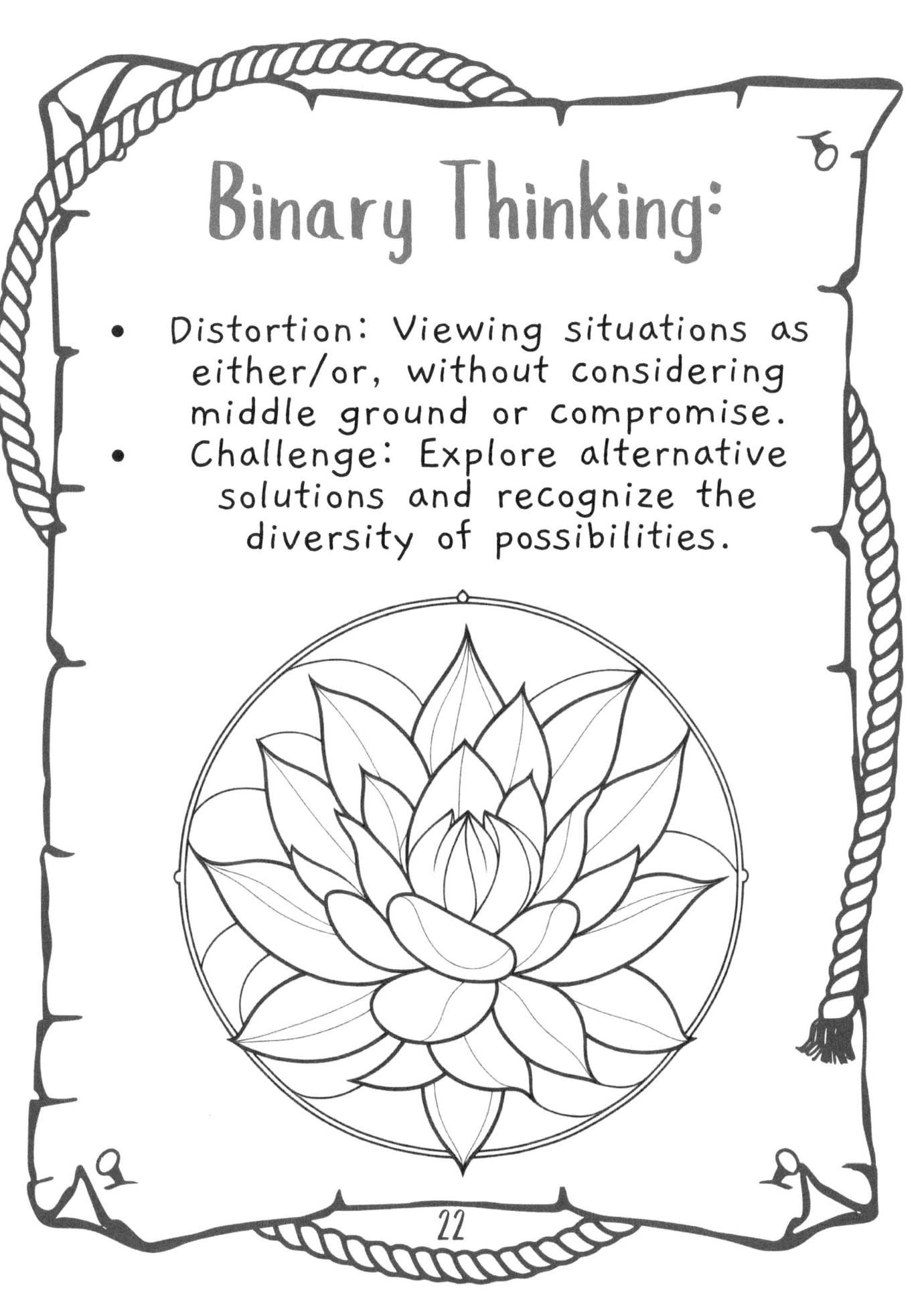

Self-Blame:

- Distortion: Holding yourself responsible for events outside your control.
- Challenge: Differentiate between responsibility and factors beyond your influence.

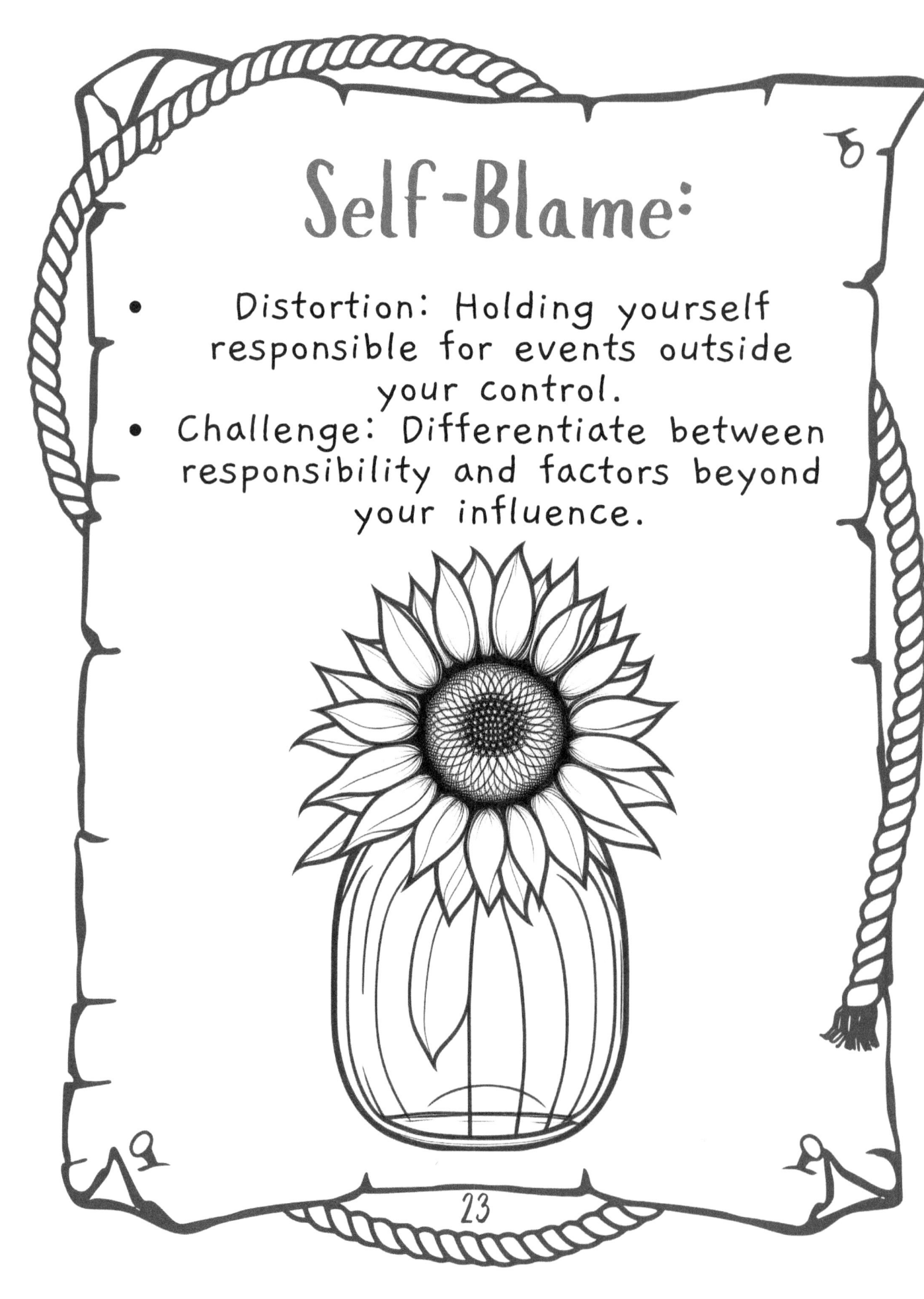

Familiarity Bias:

- Distortion: Preferring the familiar, even if it's negative, over the uncertainty of the unknown.
- Challenge: Embrace change and new experiences, recognizing their potential for growth.

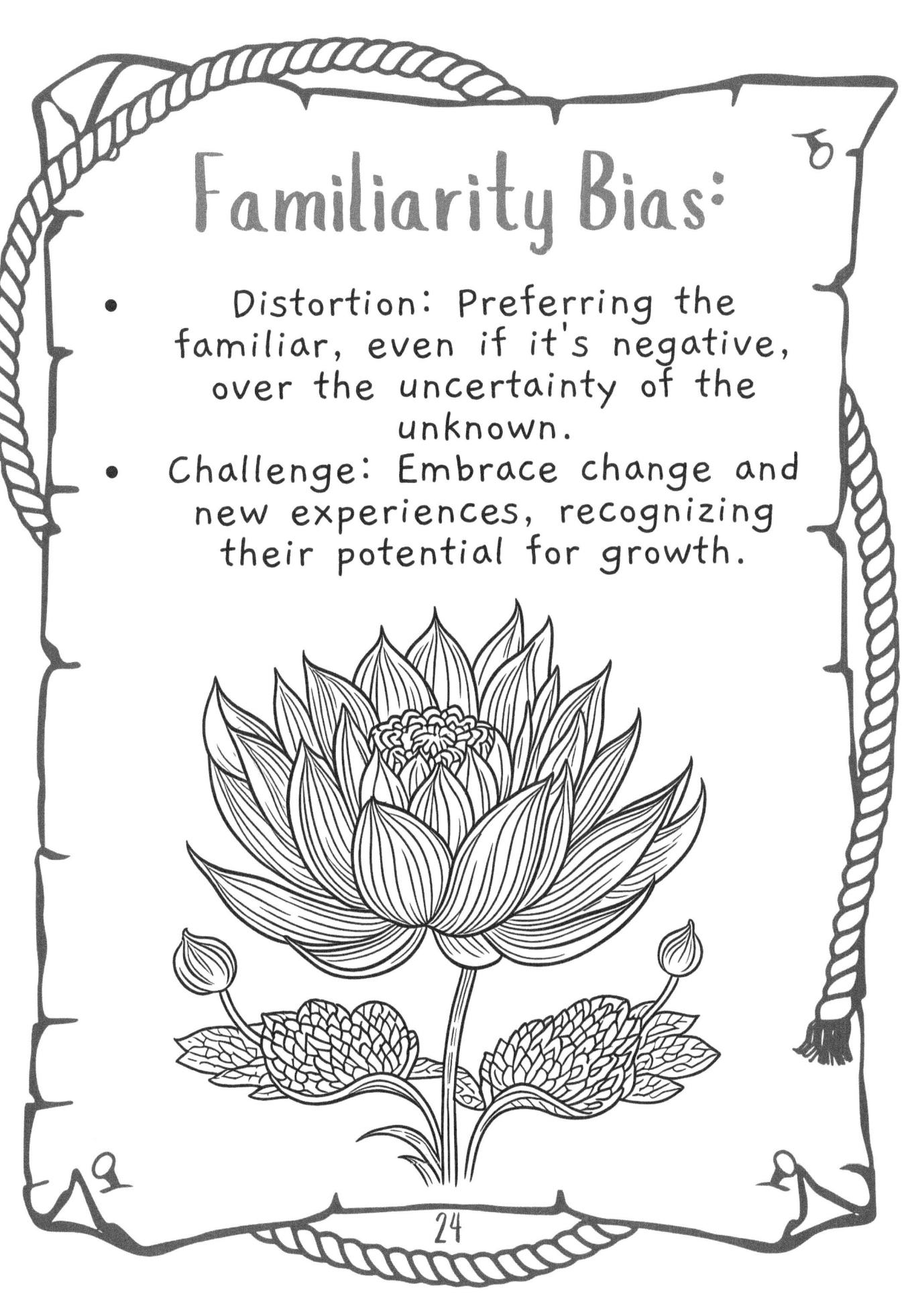

Temporal Discounting:

- Distortion: Devaluing future rewards in favor of immediate gratification.
- Challenge: Consider the long-term consequences of your actions and make decisions with future well-being in mind.

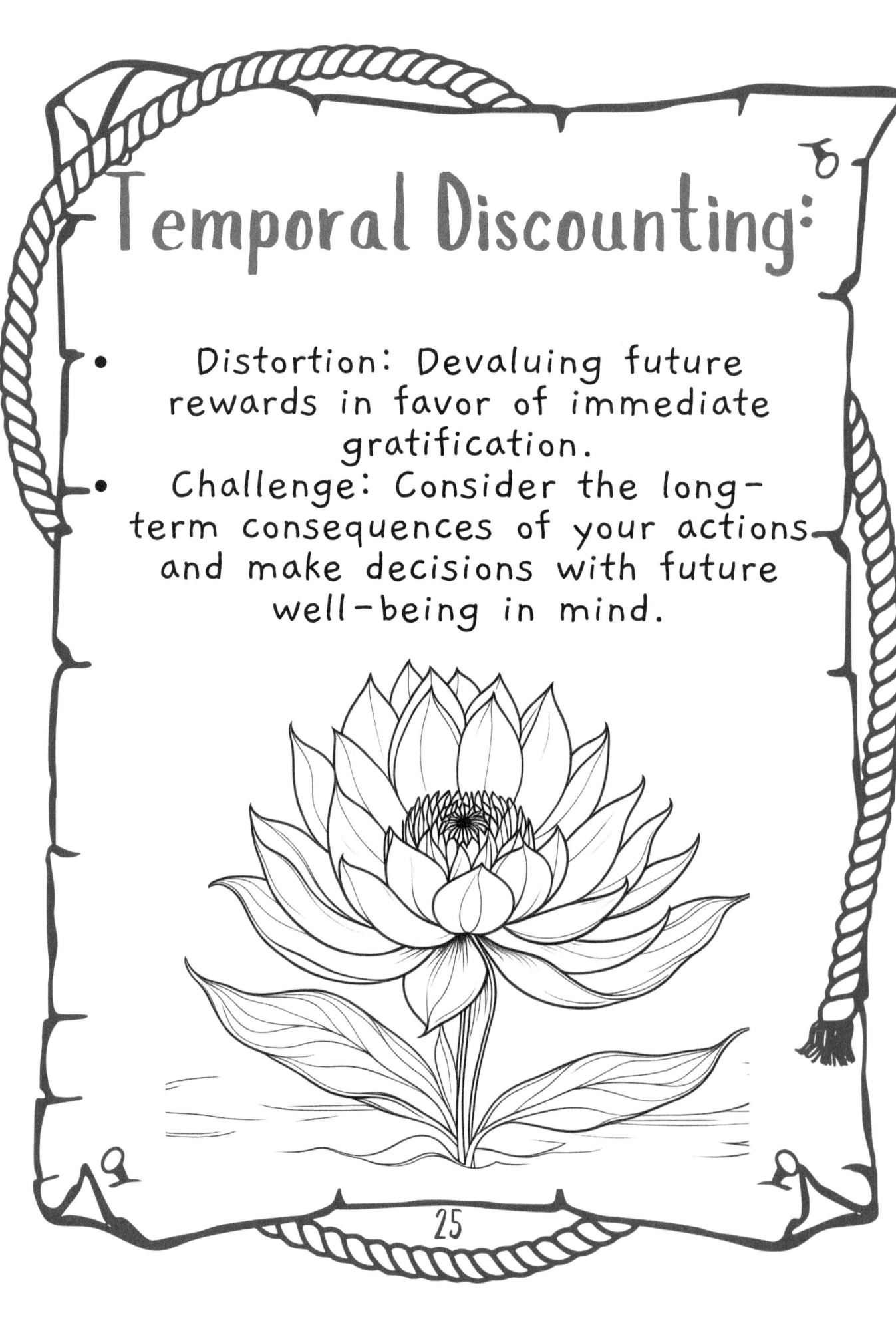

Comparative Suffering:

- Distortion: Minimizing your struggles by comparing them to others who seem worse off.
- Challenge: Acknowledge and validate your own challenges without diminishing their significance.

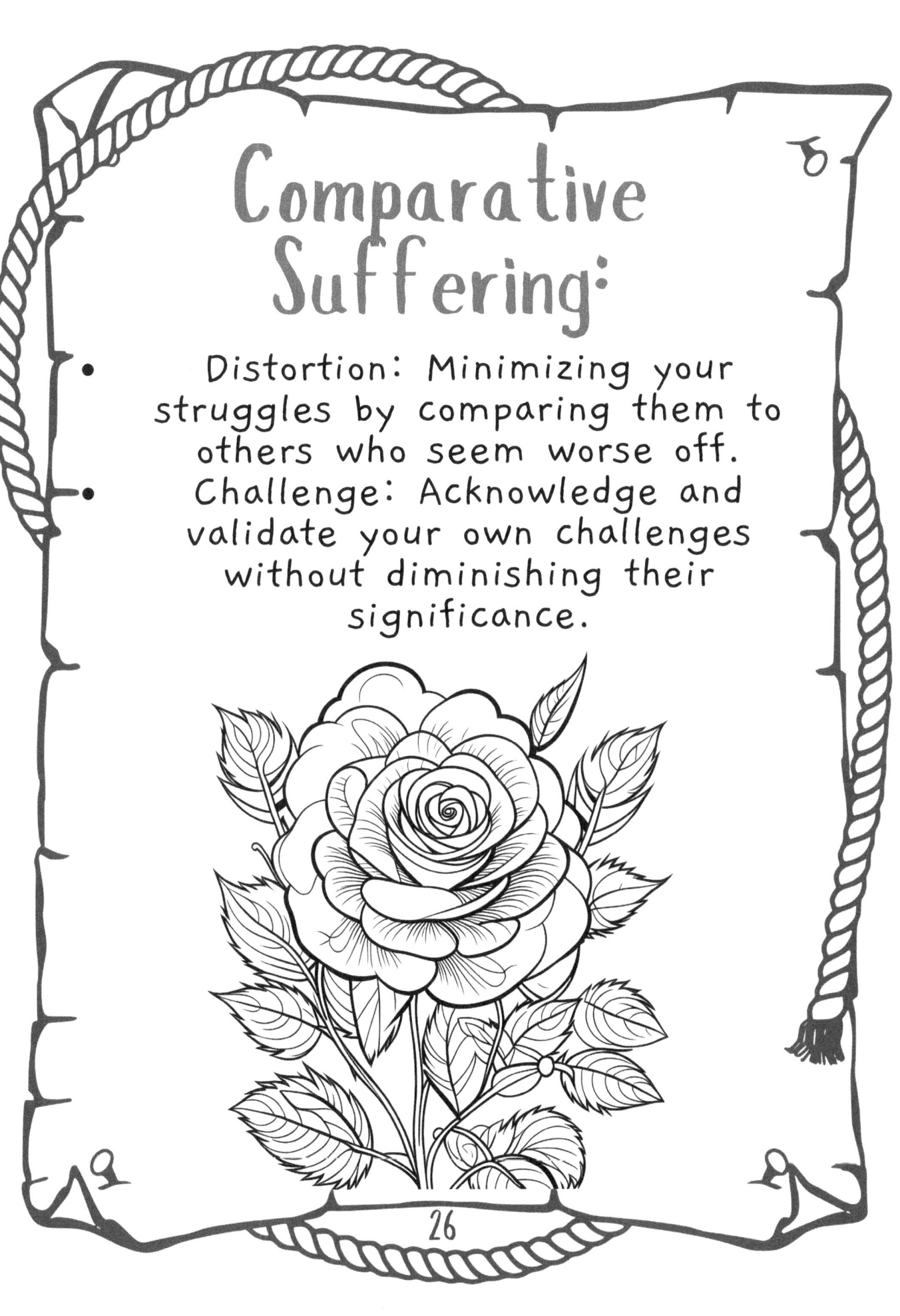

Imposter Syndrome:

- Distortion: Feeling inadequate despite evidence of competence.
- Challenge: Recognize your accomplishments and attribute them to your skills and efforts.

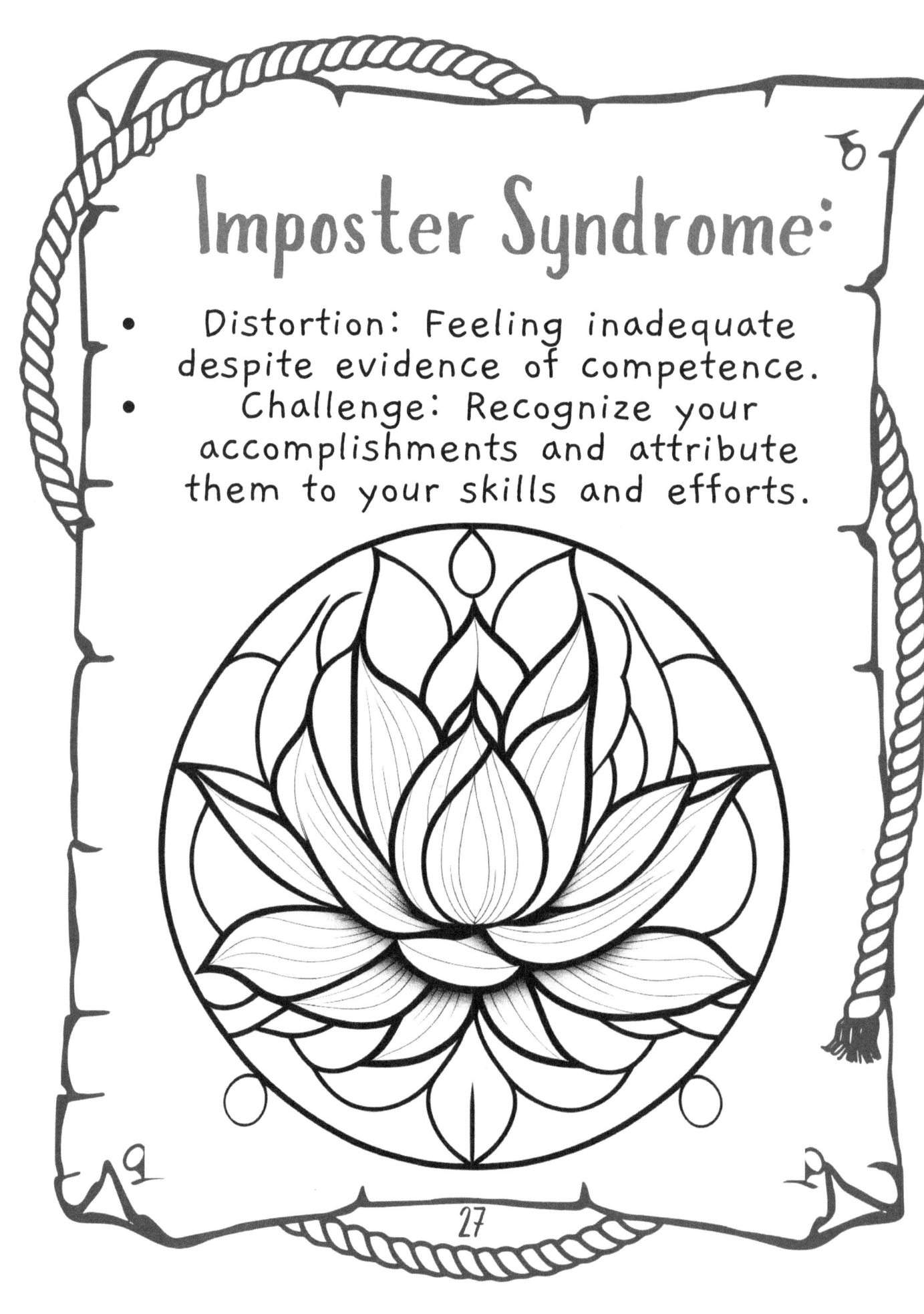

Entitlement Thinking:

- Distortion: Believing you deserve special treatment without earning it.
- Challenge: Cultivate a mindset of earning rewards through effort and merit.

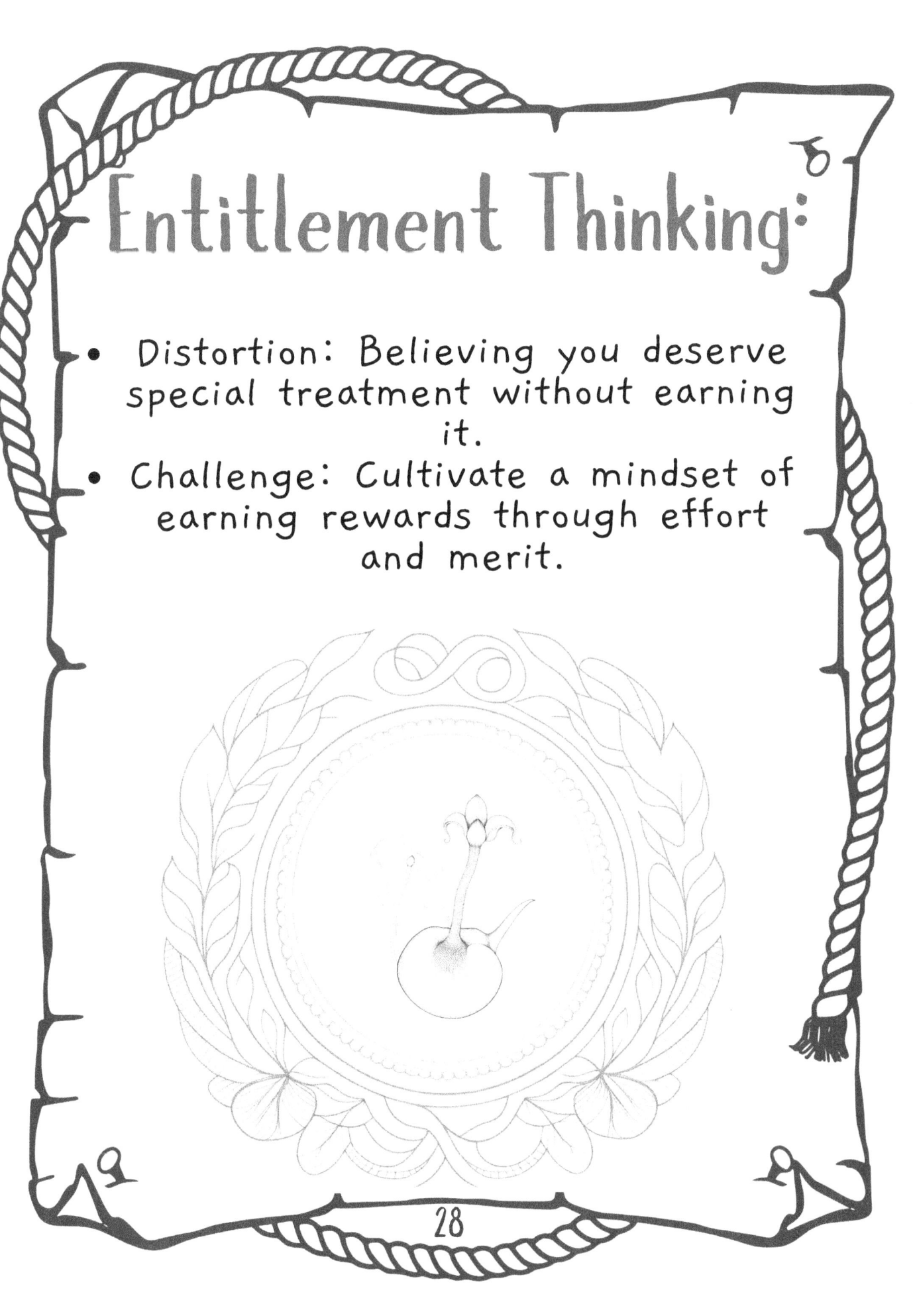

Perfectionism:

- Distortion: Setting unrealistically high standards and feeling a constant need to meet them.
- Challenge: Embrace the concept of "good enough" and appreciate the value of progress over perfection.

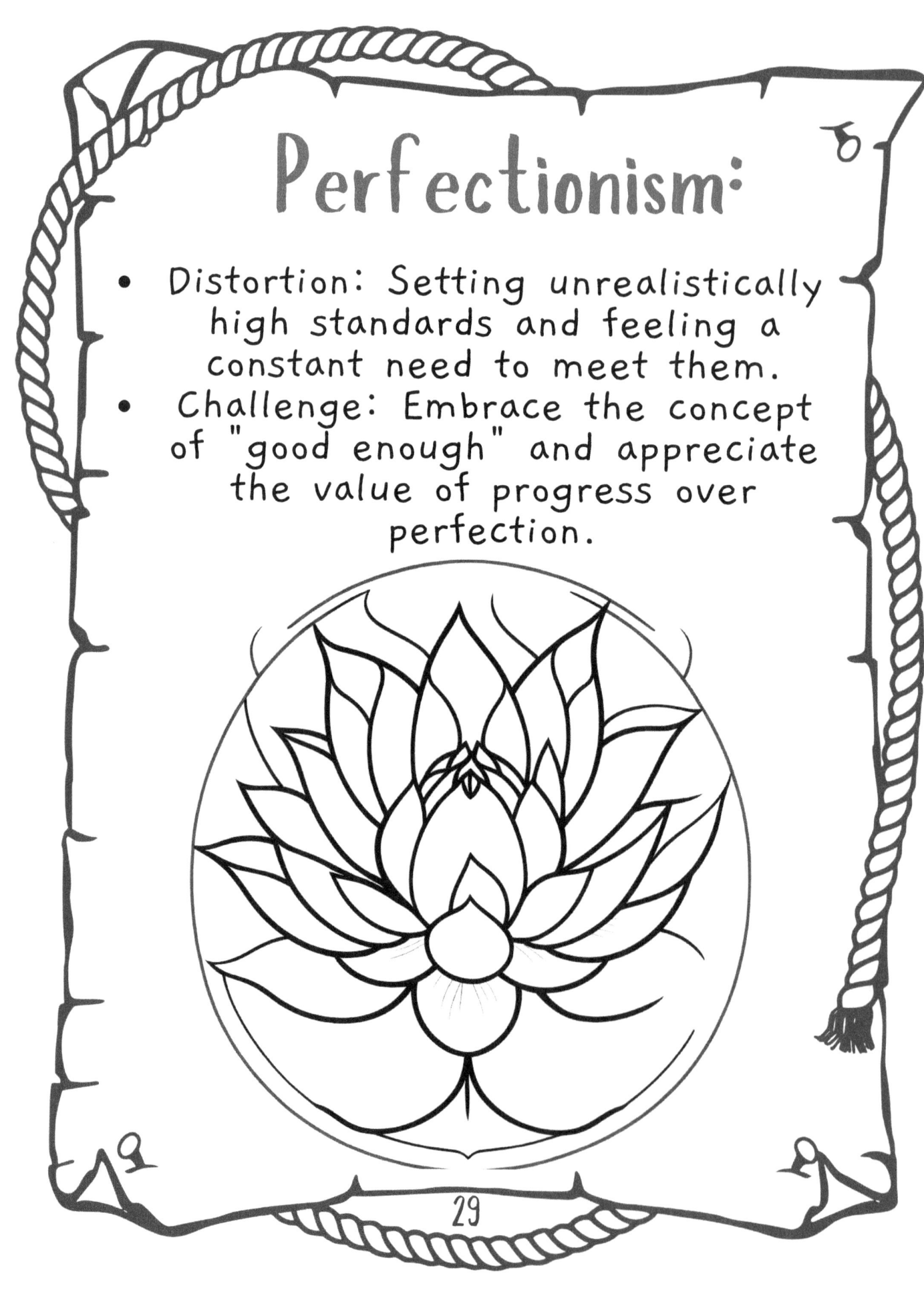

Victim Mentality:

- Distortion: Seeing oneself as a perpetual victim, blaming external factors for personal challenges.
- Challenge: Take ownership of your choices and focus on solutions rather than dwelling on problems.

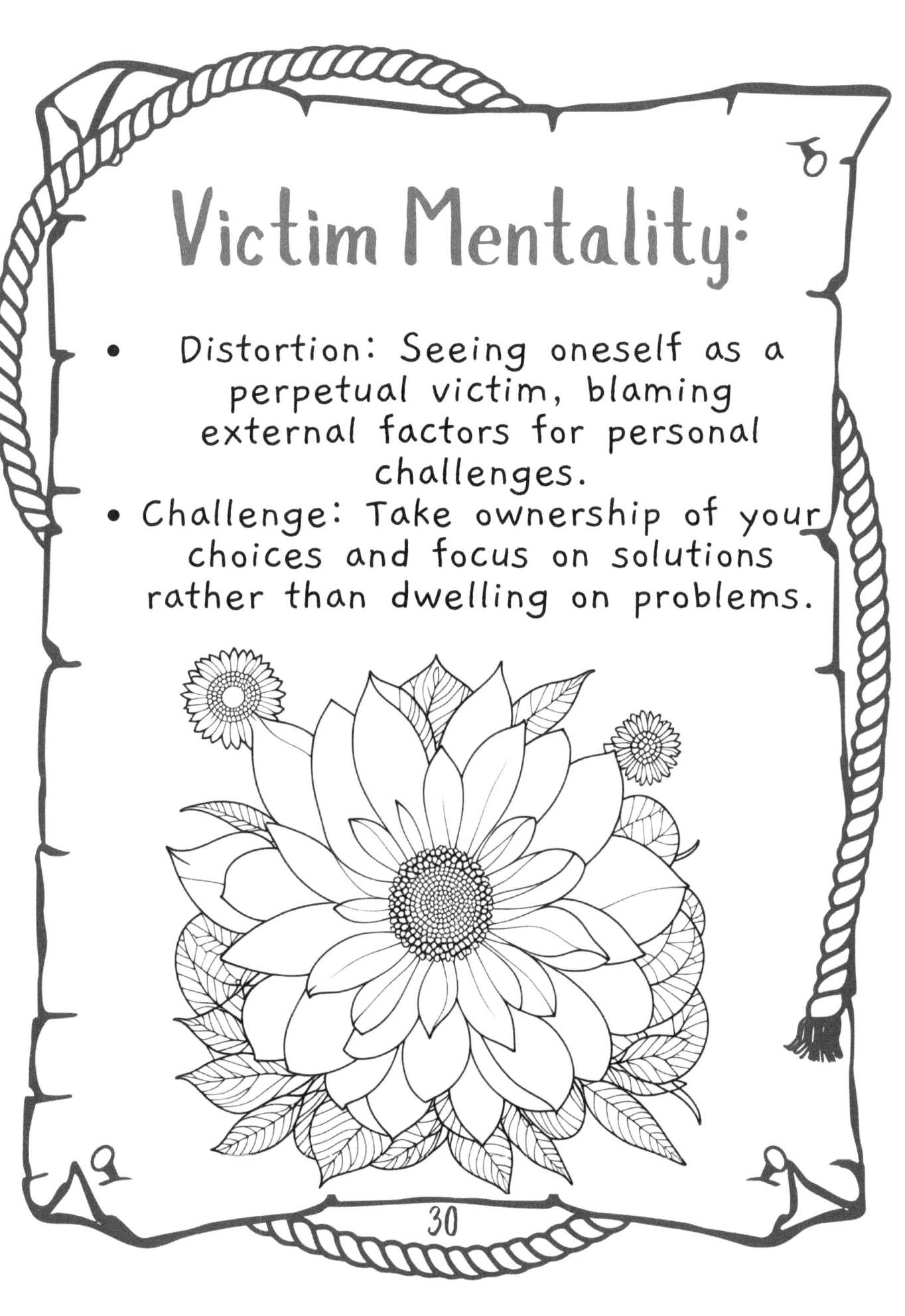

Selective Memory:

- Distortion: Recalling only information that supports negative beliefs.
- Challenge: Actively seek out and remember positive experiences to balance your perspective.

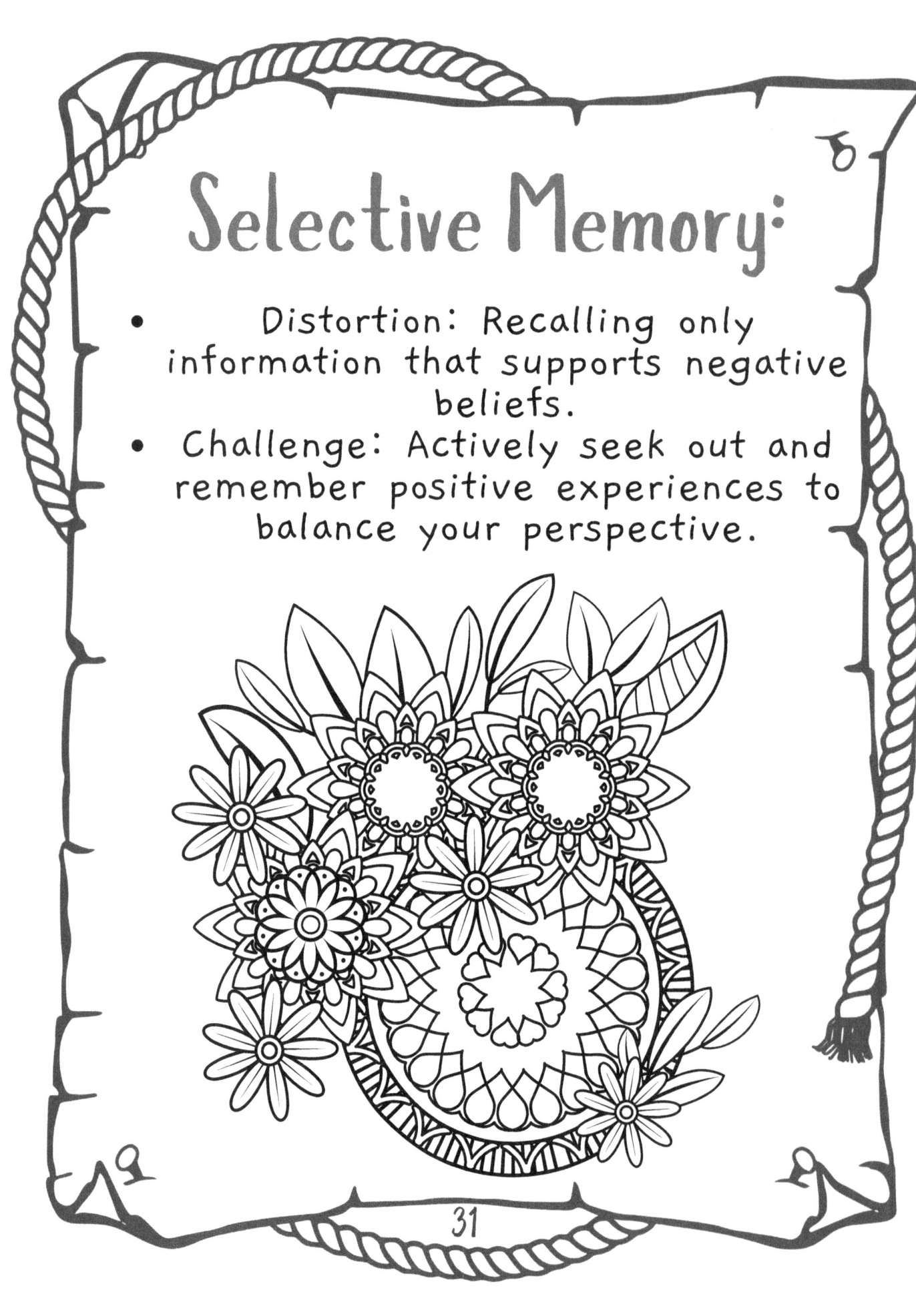

Social Comparison Trap:

- Distortion: Constantly measuring your worth against others, leading to feelings of inadequacy.
- Challenge: Recognize that everyone has their unique journey and focus on personal growth instead of comparison.

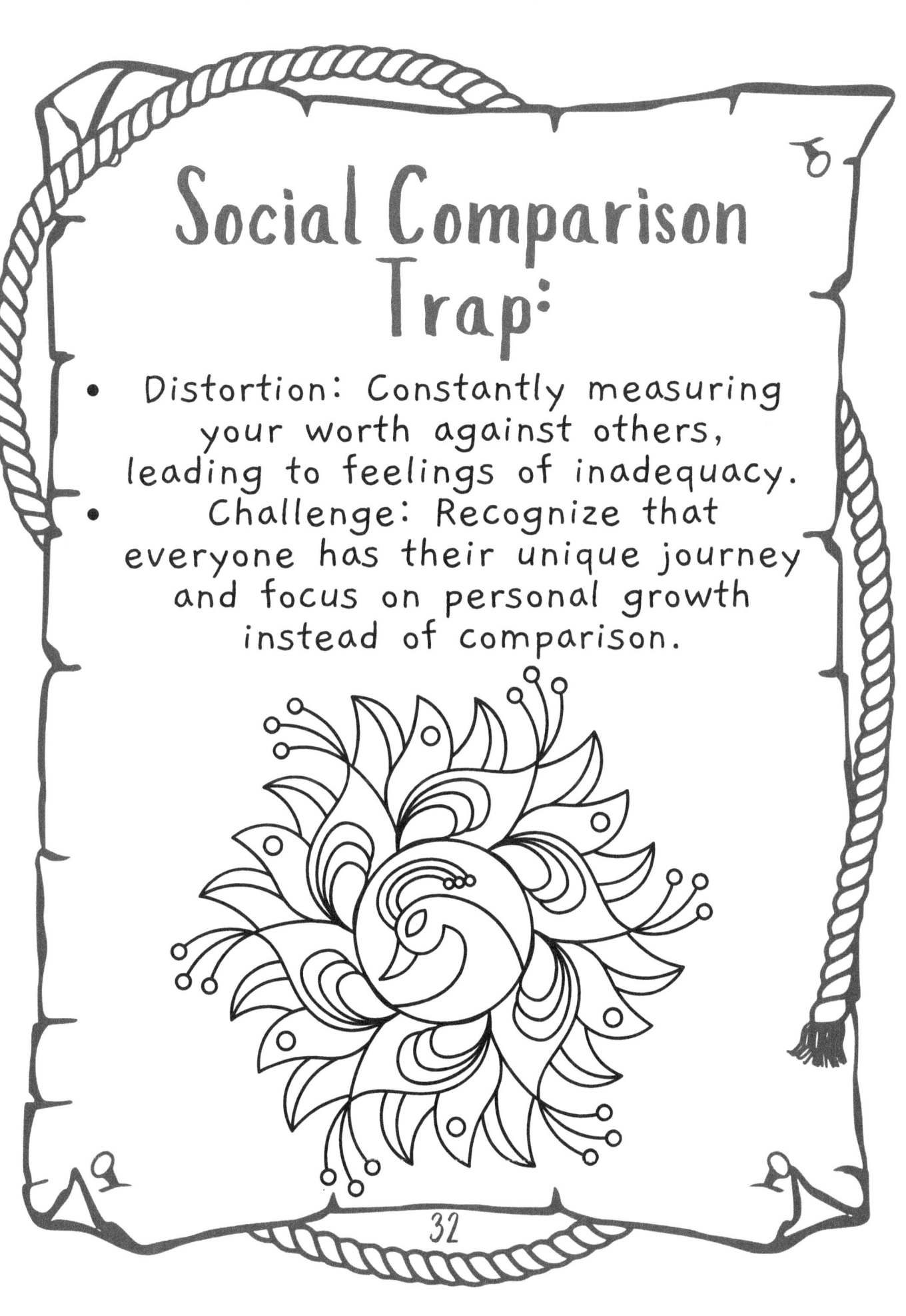

Fear of Rejection:

- Distortion: Anticipating rejection and avoiding situations that might involve it.
- Challenge: Approach social interactions with an open mind, acknowledging that rejection is a natural part of life.

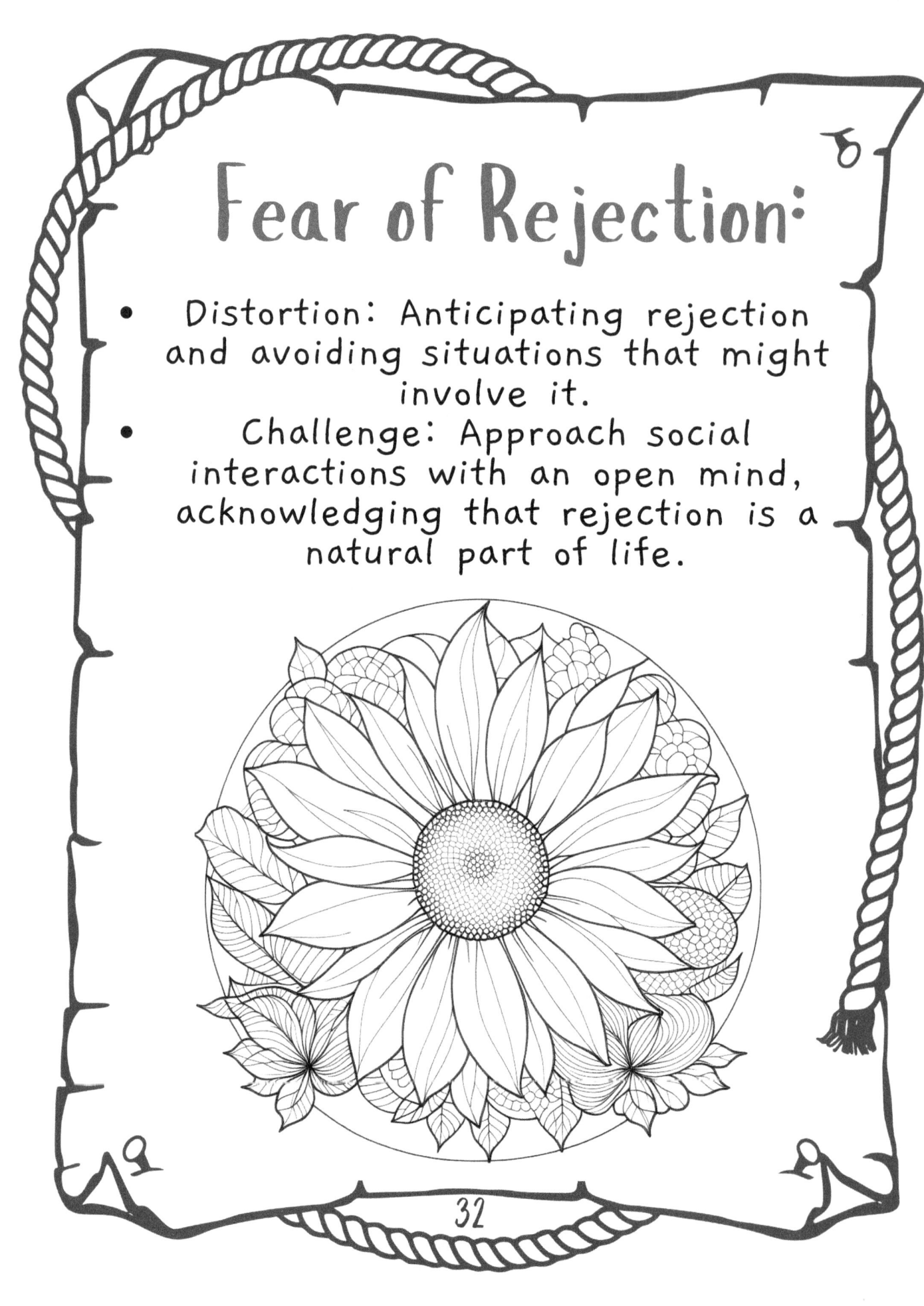

Overpersonalization:

- Distortion: Taking things personally, even when they have little to do with you.
- Challenge: Consider alternative explanations for others' behavior and avoid assuming everything is about you.

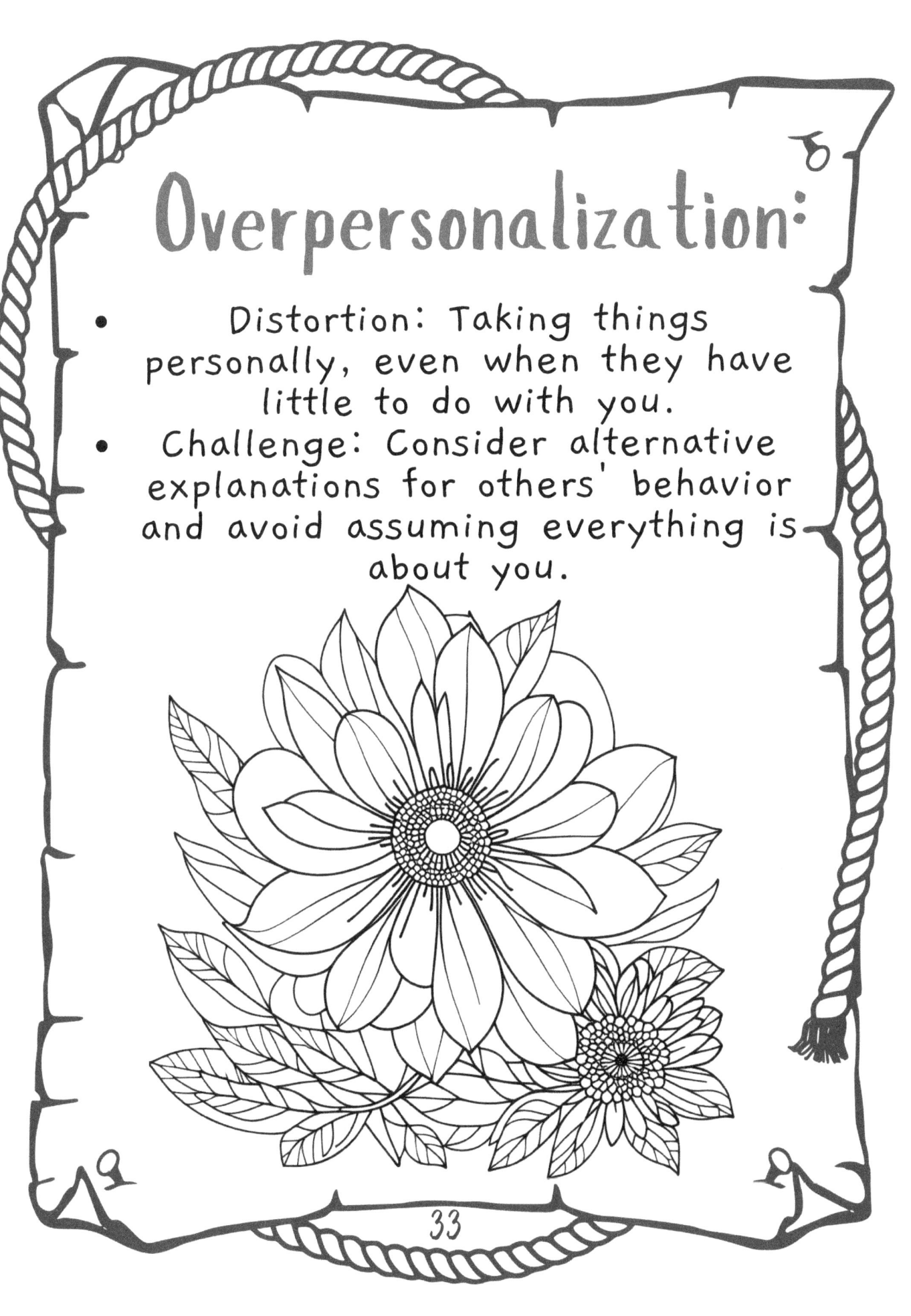

Rumination:

- Distortion: Getting stuck in negative thought patterns, replaying and overanalyzing past events.
- Challenge: Practice mindfulness techniques to stay present and break the cycle of rumination.

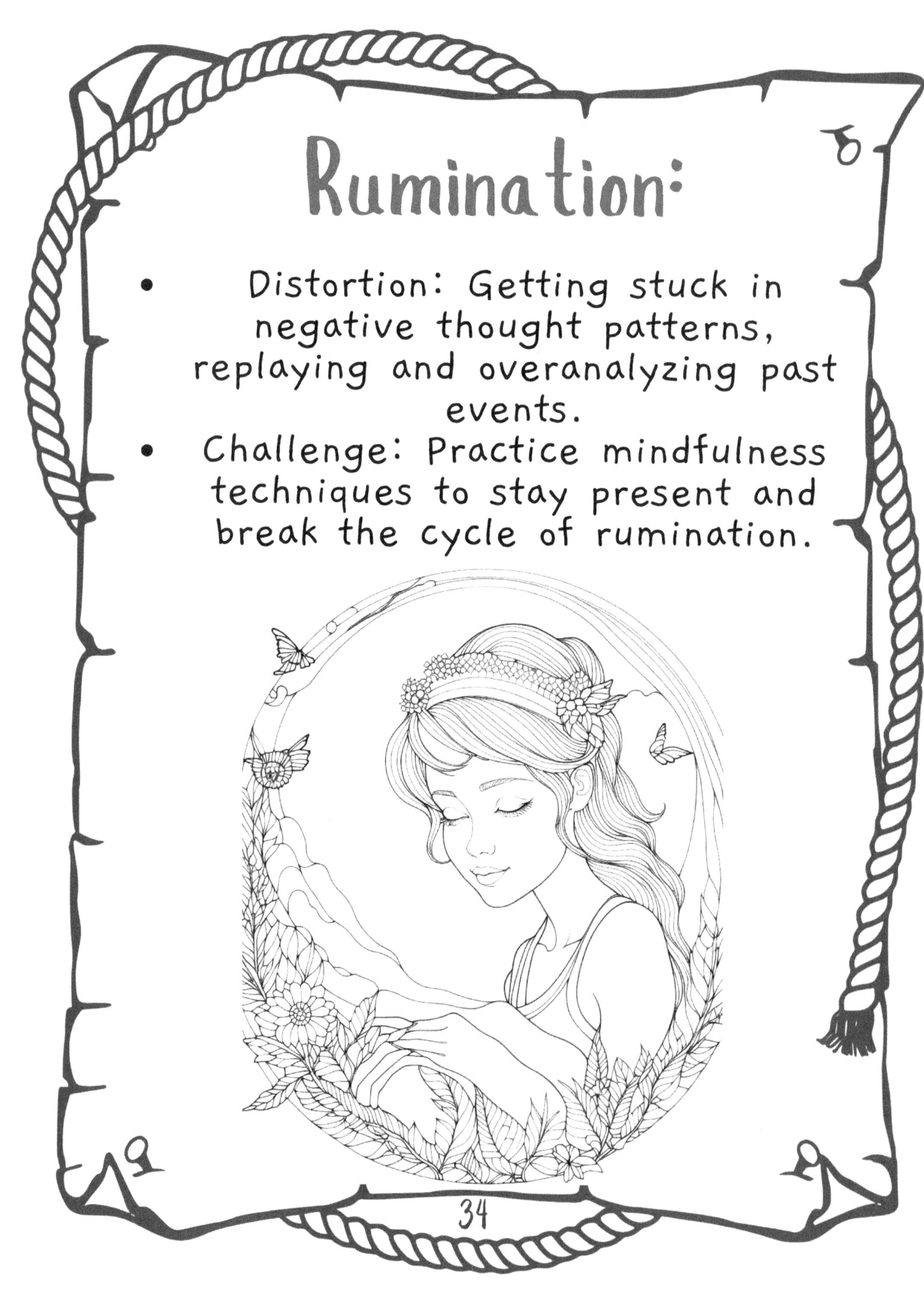

Neglecting Positives in Relationships:

- Distortion: Focusing on the flaws and shortcomings in relationships while overlooking positive aspects.
- Challenge: Regularly express gratitude and appreciate the positive qualities in your relationships.

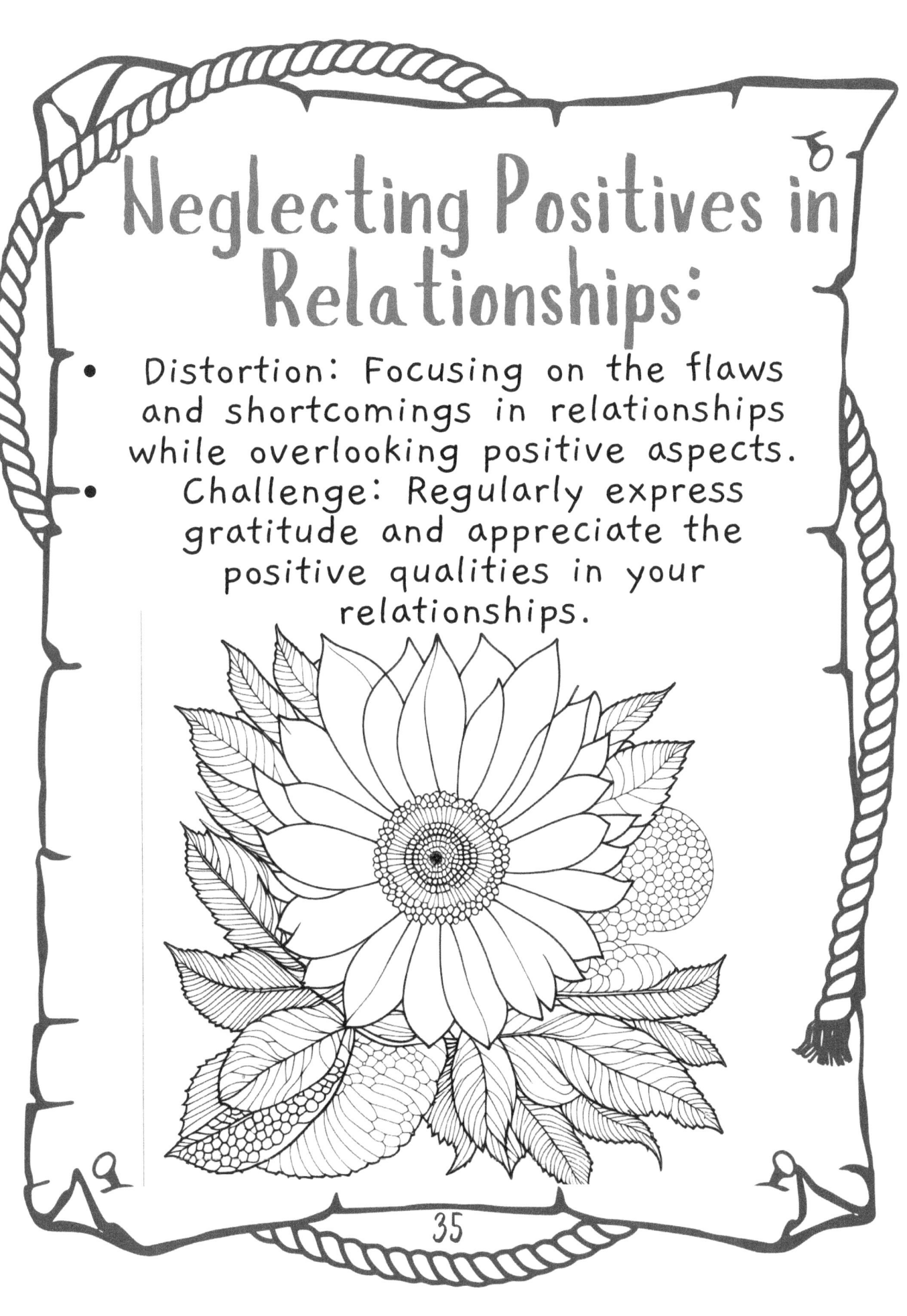

Comparing Internal Feelings to External Appearances:

- Distortion: Assuming others have it all together based on outward appearances.
- Challenge: Remember that everyone faces challenges, and external appearances may not reflect internal struggles.

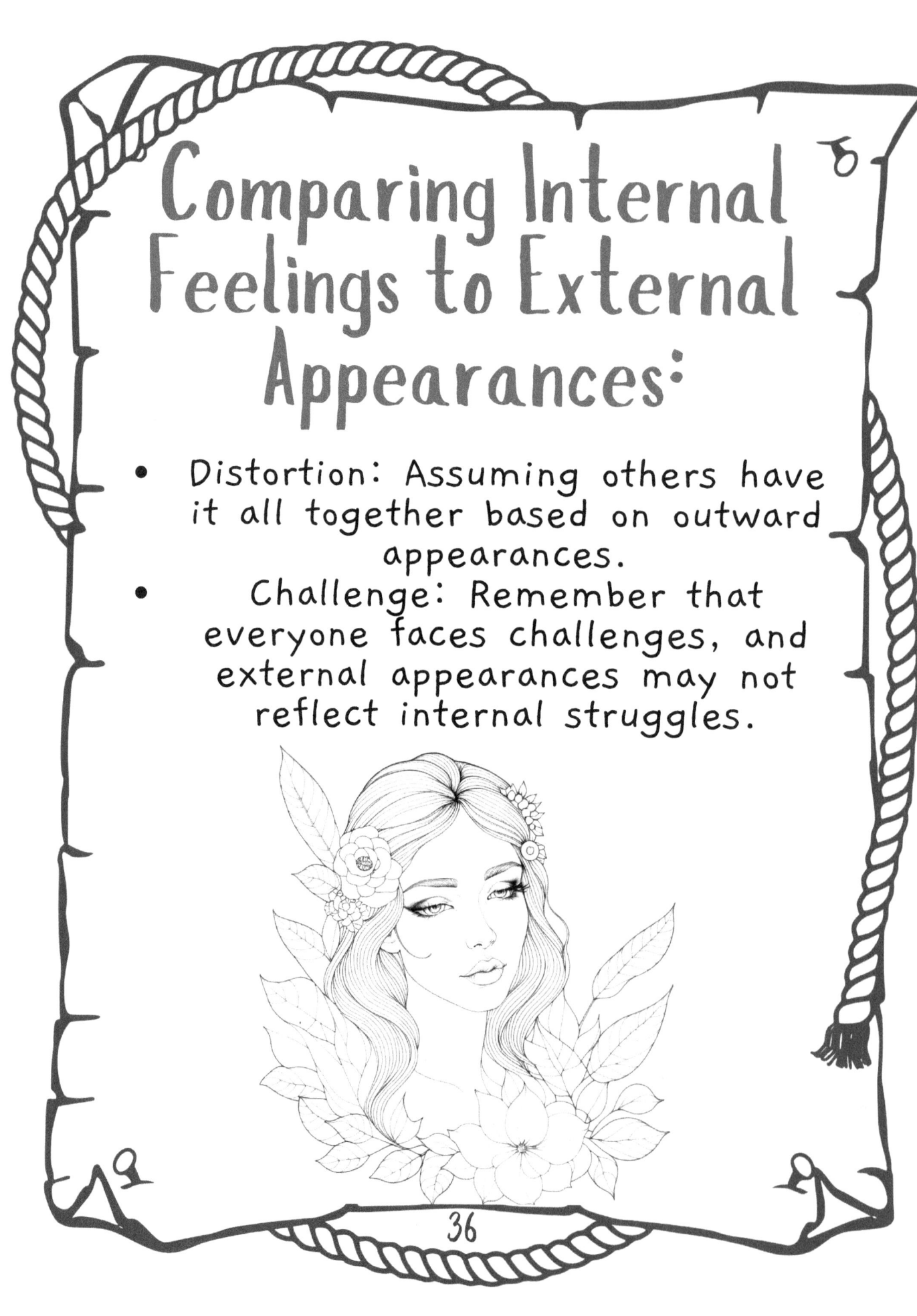

Overestimating Future Discomfort:

- Distortion: Expecting future events to be more distressing than they are likely to be.
- Challenge: Approach new experiences with an open mind, recognizing that discomfort is a natural part of growth.

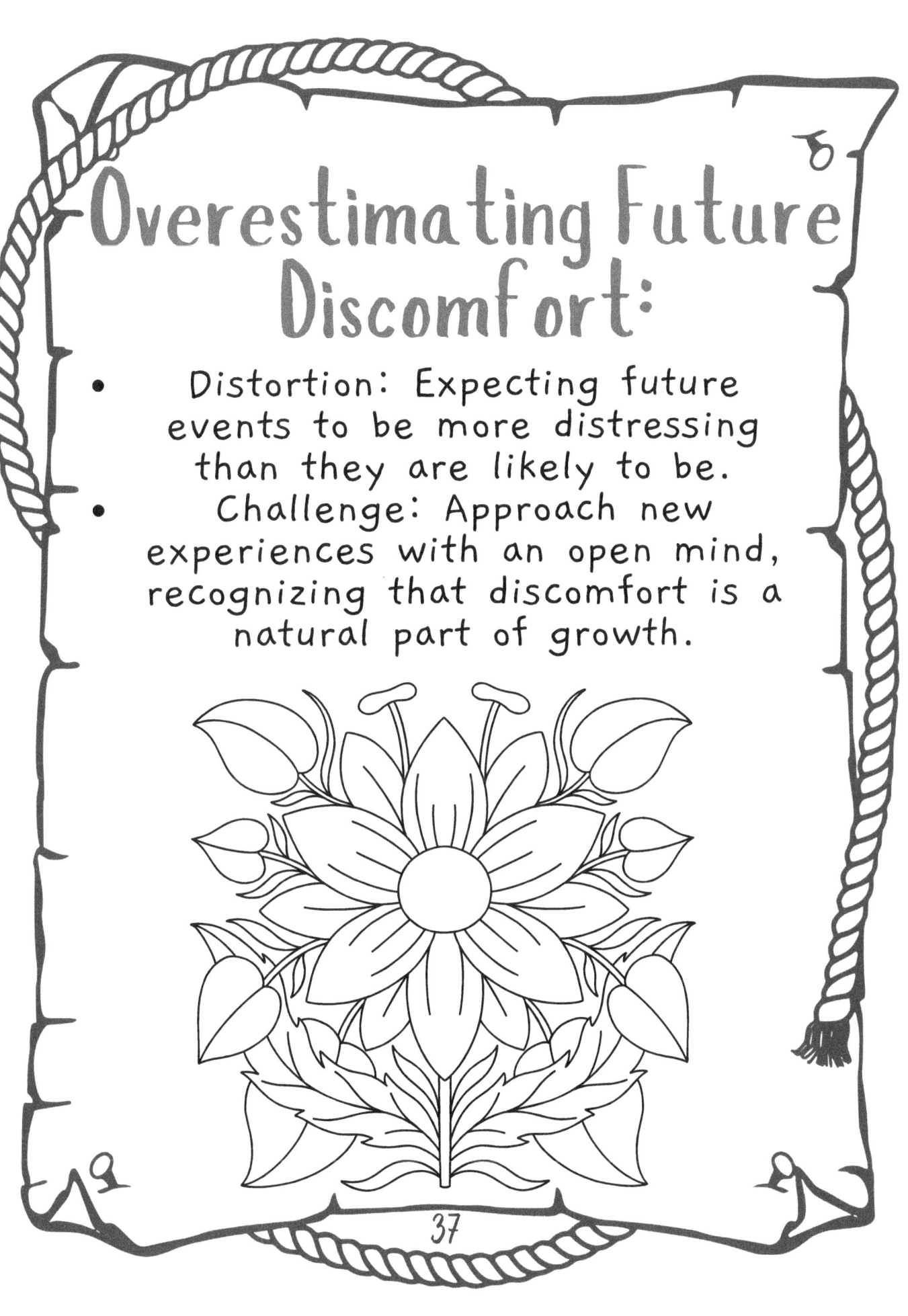

Minimizing Achievements:

- Distortion: Dismissing your accomplishments as insignificant or attributing them to luck.
- Challenge: Take pride in your achievements and acknowledge the effort and skill that contributed to them.

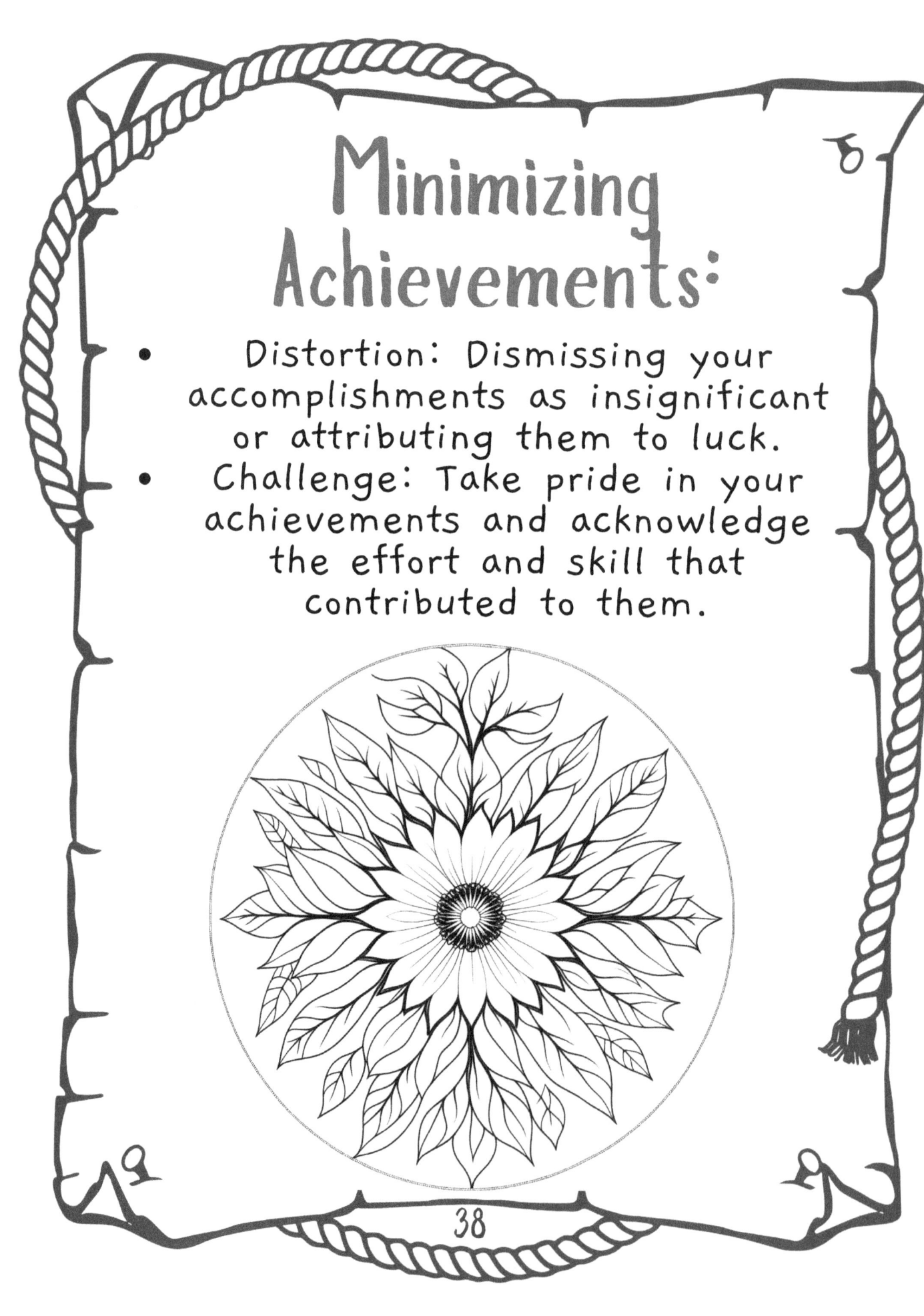

Discounting Feedback:

- Distortion: Dismissing positive feedback and focusing only on criticism.
- Challenge: Accept and internalize positive feedback, recognizing your strengths and abilities.

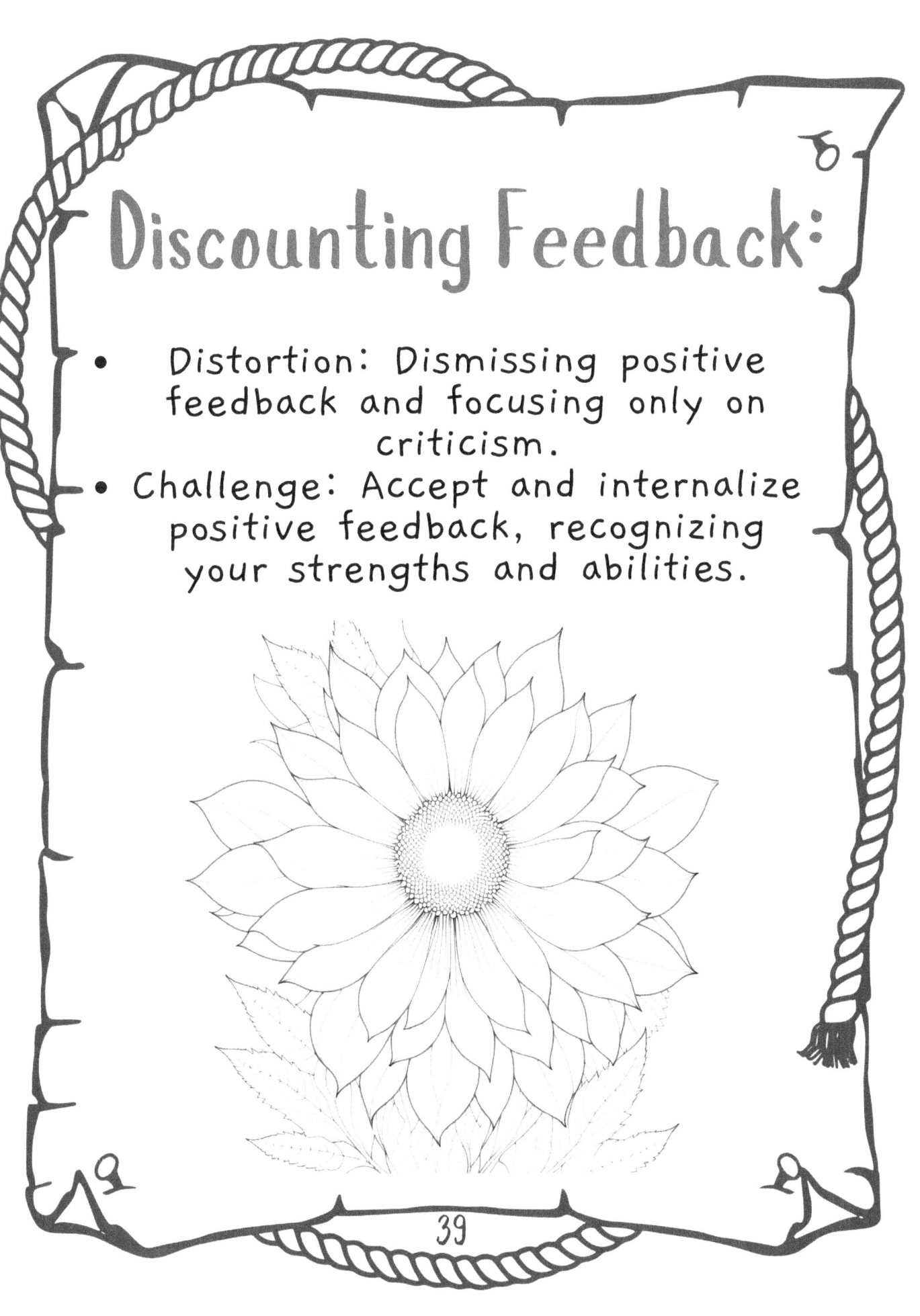

Cognitive Tunneling:

- Distortion: Fixating on a single negative detail and losing sight of the bigger picture.
- Challenge: Broaden your perspective by consciously seeking out positive aspects and alternative viewpoints.

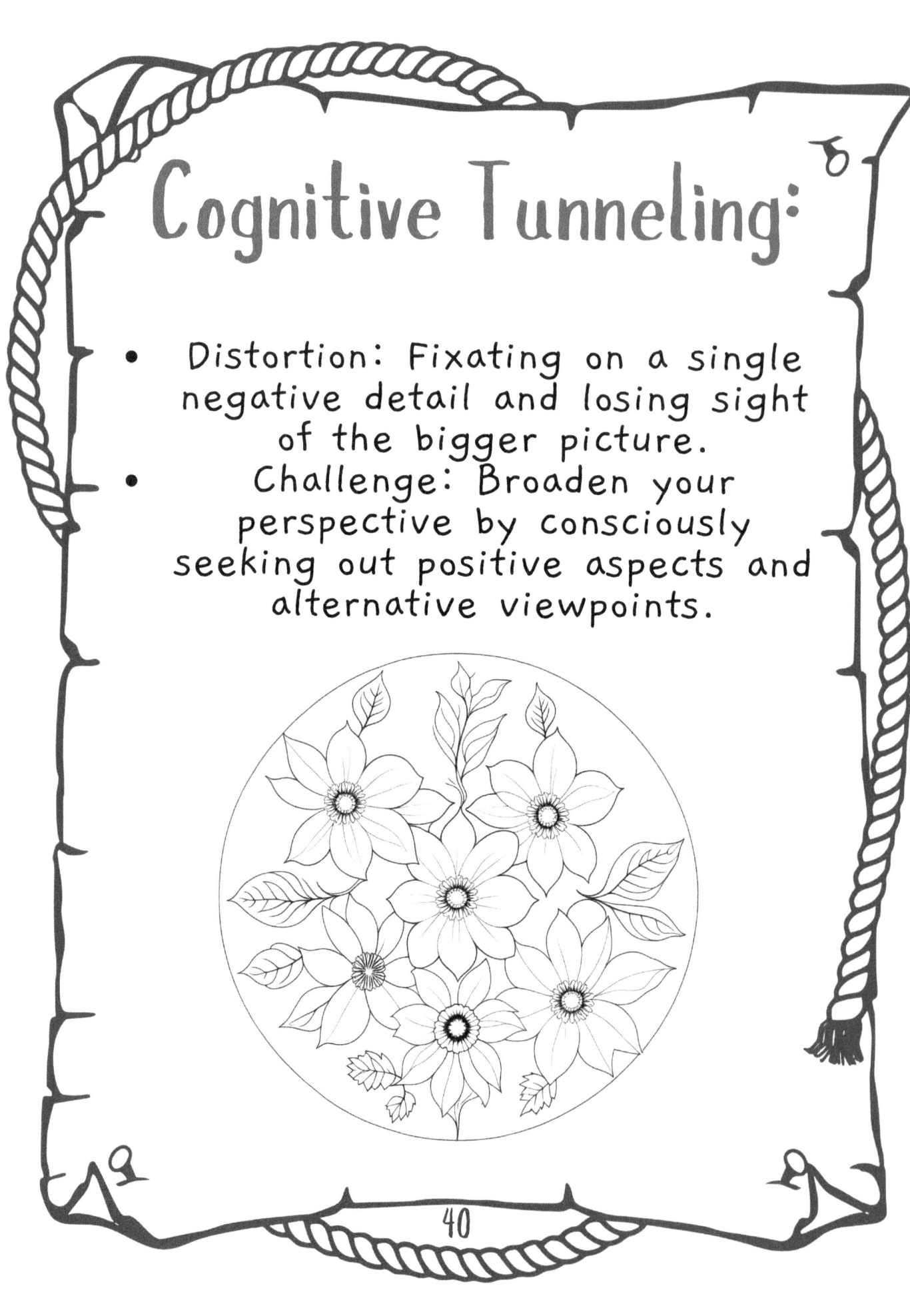

Escalation of Commitment:

- Distortion: Persisting in a course of action despite negative outcomes, simply because you've invested time or effort.
- Challenge: Evaluate situations objectively and be willing to adapt or change course when necessary.

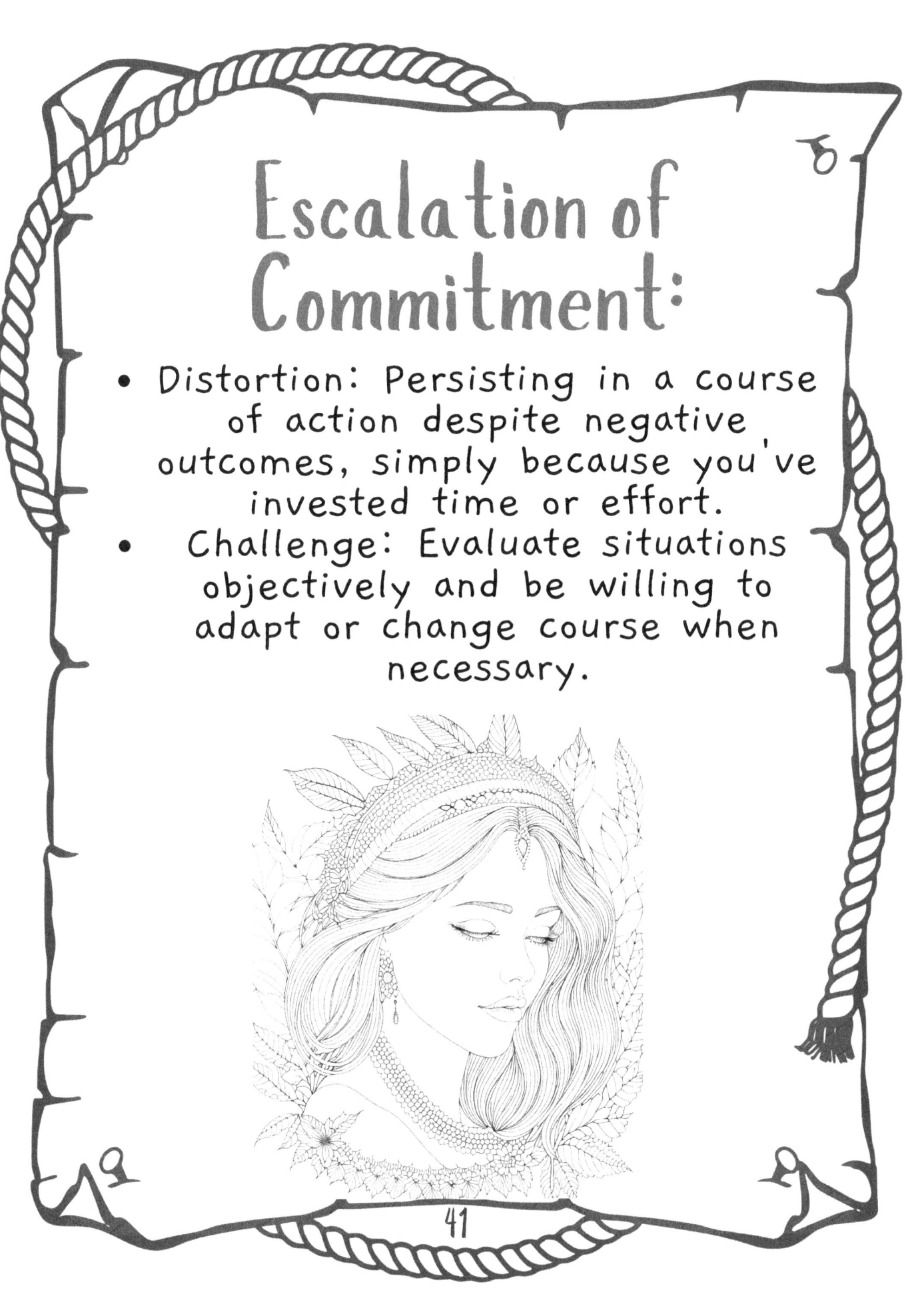

Shouldering the Burden of Others:

- Distortion: Taking on responsibility for other people's problems.
- Challenge: Offer support when appropriate, but recognize and respect others' agency in solving their issues.

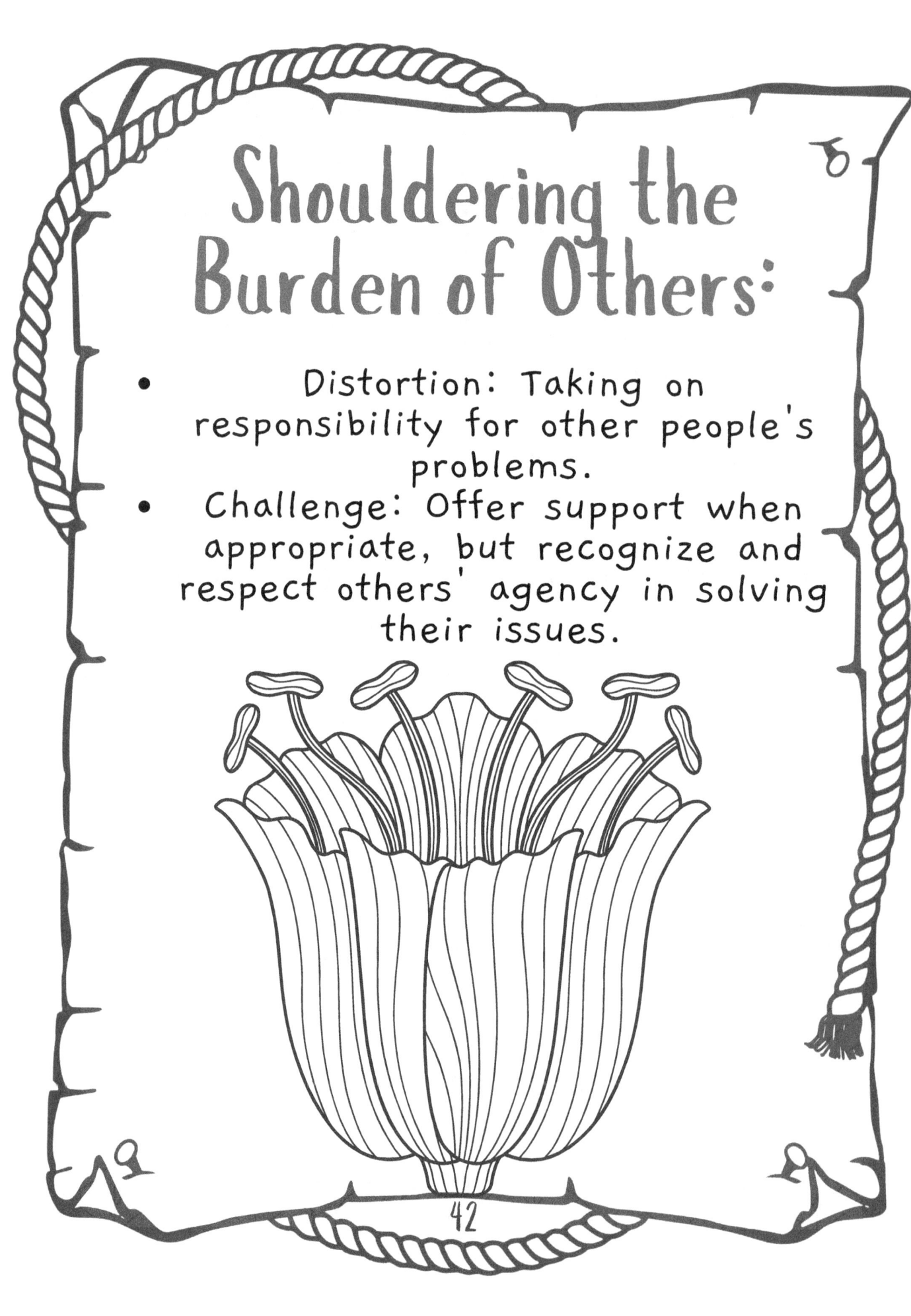

Fatalism:

- Distortion: Believing that events are predetermined and beyond your control.
- Challenge: Take an active role in shaping your destiny; focus on what you can influence.

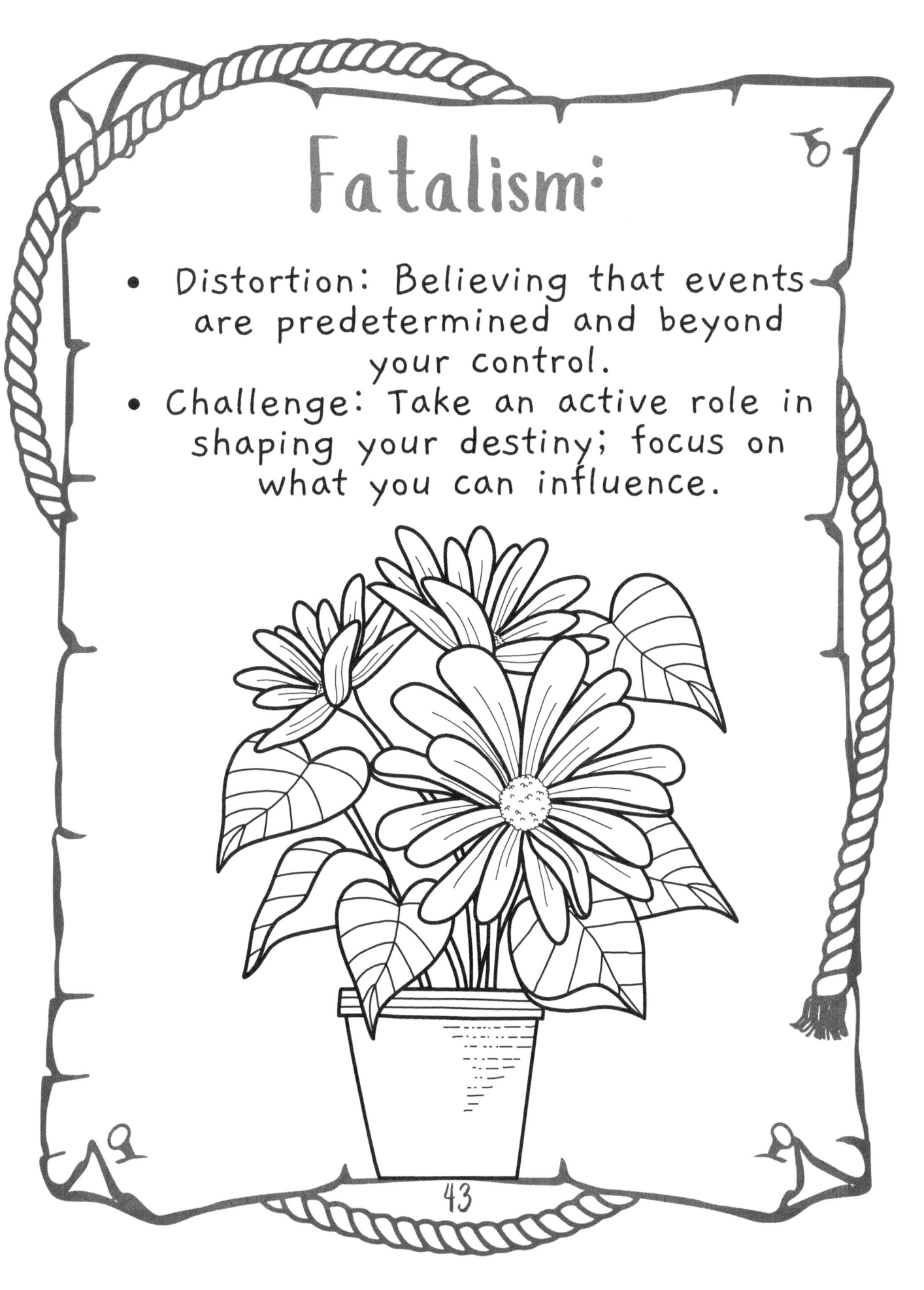

Polarized Thinking in Relationships:

- Distortion: Seeing relationships as either perfect or a complete failure.
- Challenge: Embrace the complexity of relationships; recognize that they evolve and require effort.

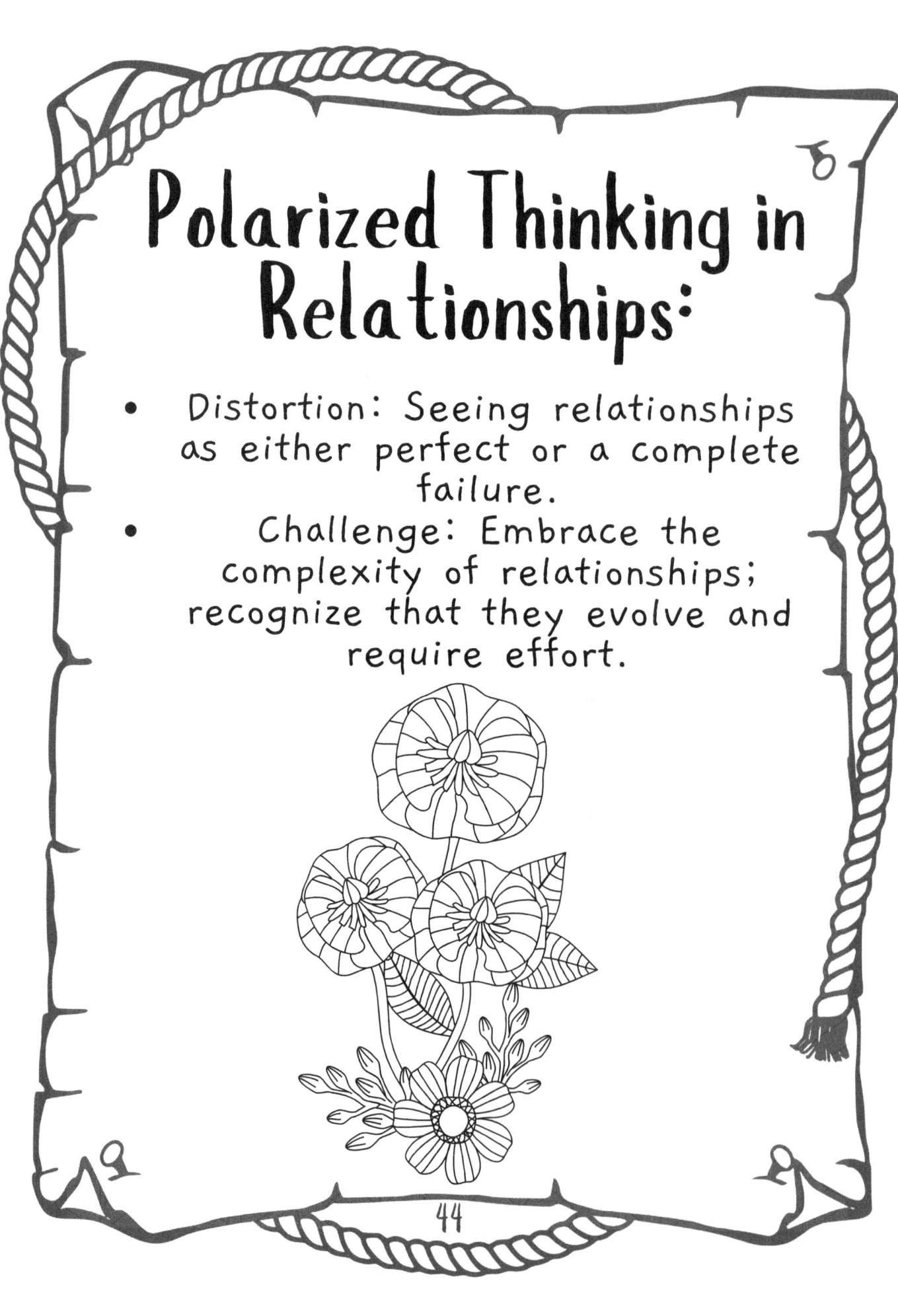

Comparing Current State to Idealized Past:

- Distortion: Idealizing the past and feeling discontent with the present.
- Challenge: Appreciate the positive aspects of the present and acknowledge the growth over time.

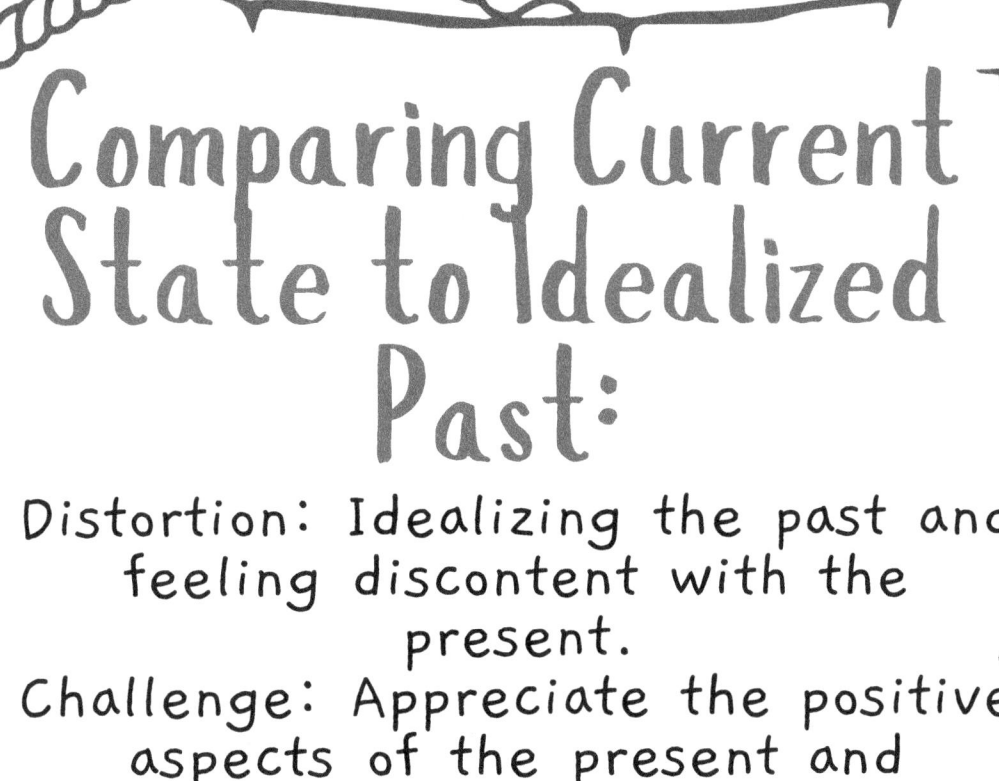

Inability to Tolerate Uncertainty:

- Distortion: Feeling unbearable distress when faced with uncertainty.
- Challenge: Build resilience by gradually exposing yourself to uncertainty, developing coping mechanisms along the way.

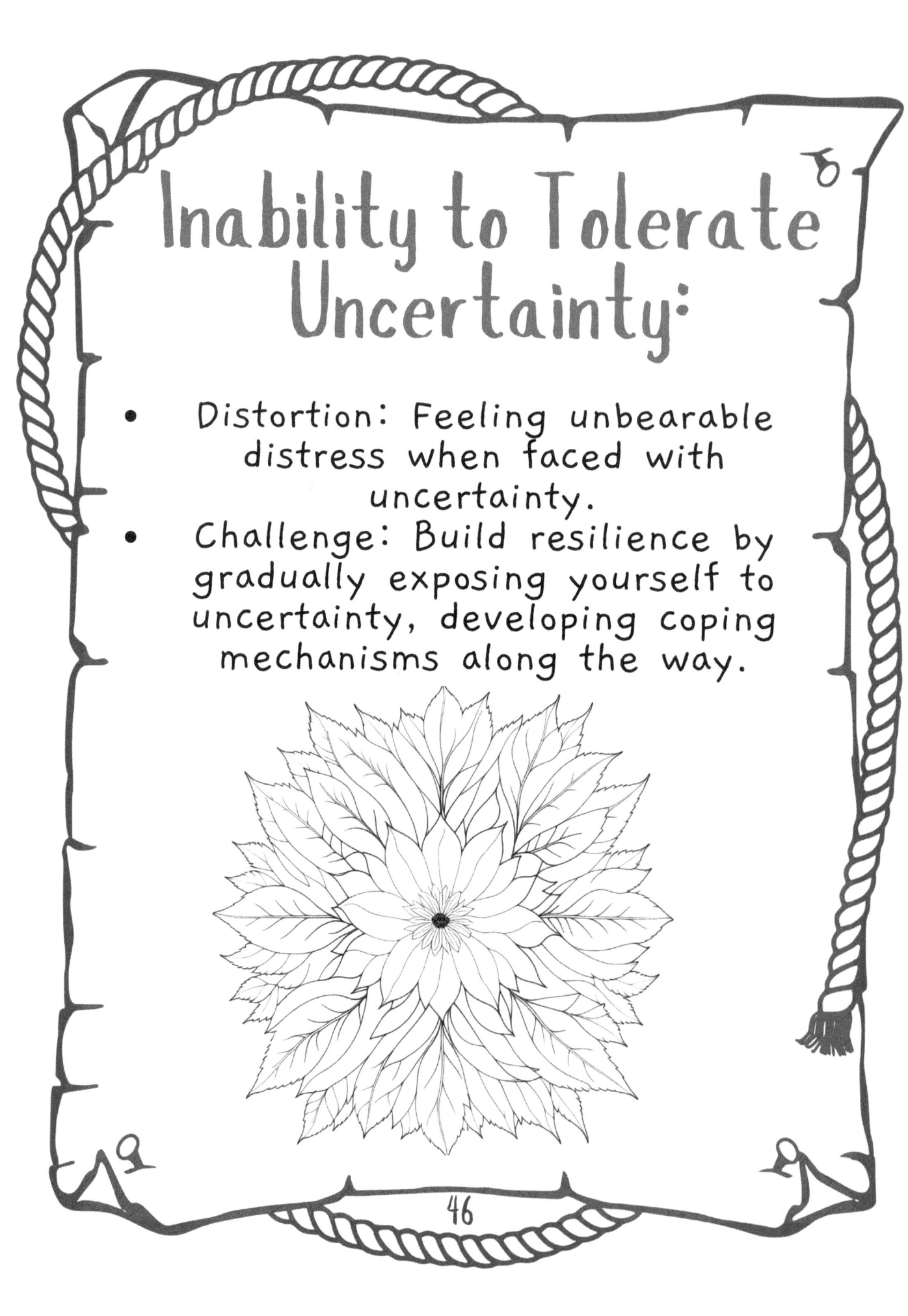

Overemphasis on Material Success:

- Distortion: Linking self-worth solely to material achievements.
- Challenge: Recognize the importance of personal growth, relationships, and well-being beyond material success.

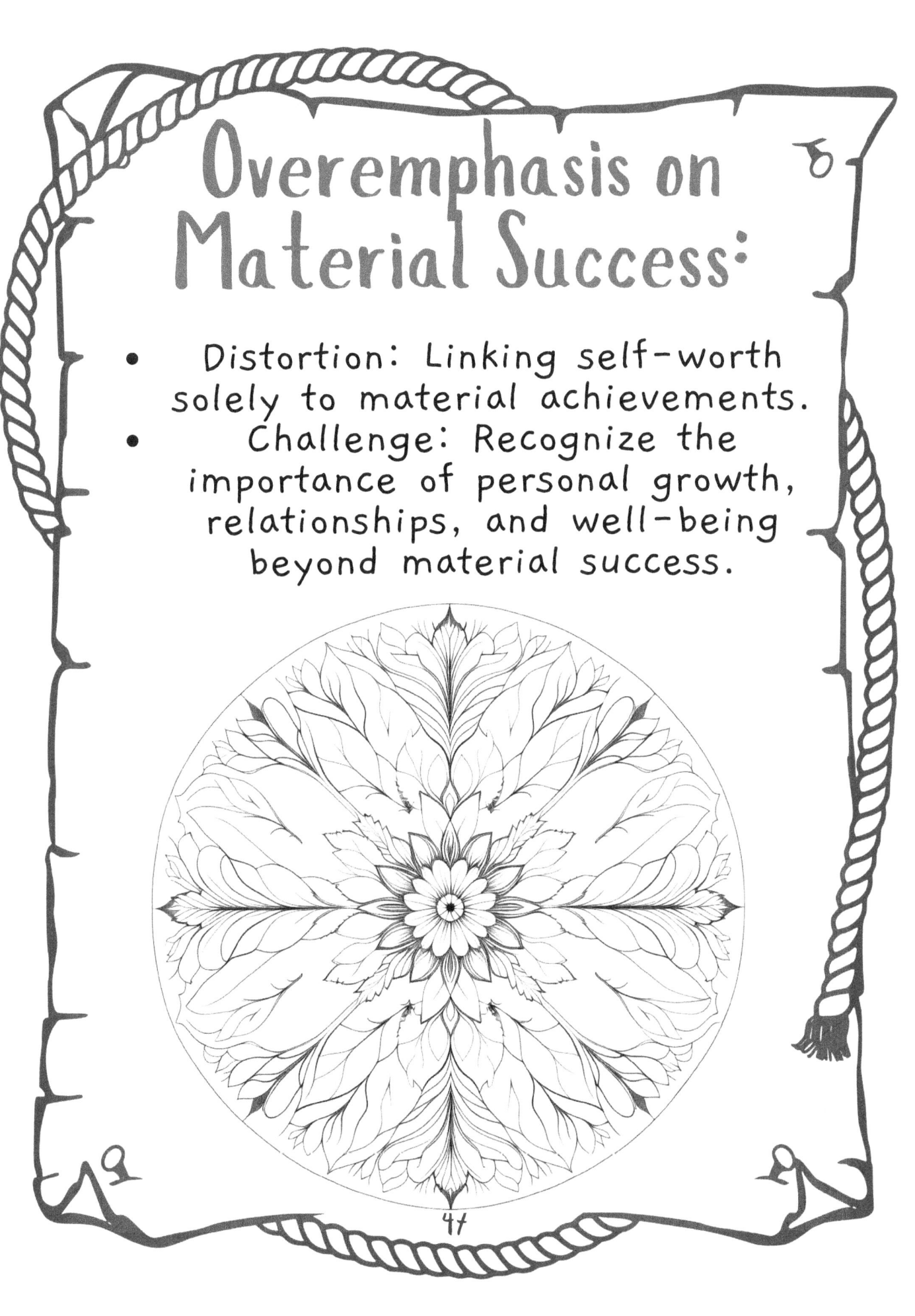

Emotional Inference:

- Distortion: Drawing conclusions about situations based on emotional states.
- Challenge: Separate emotions from facts, allowing for a more rational assessment of circumstances.

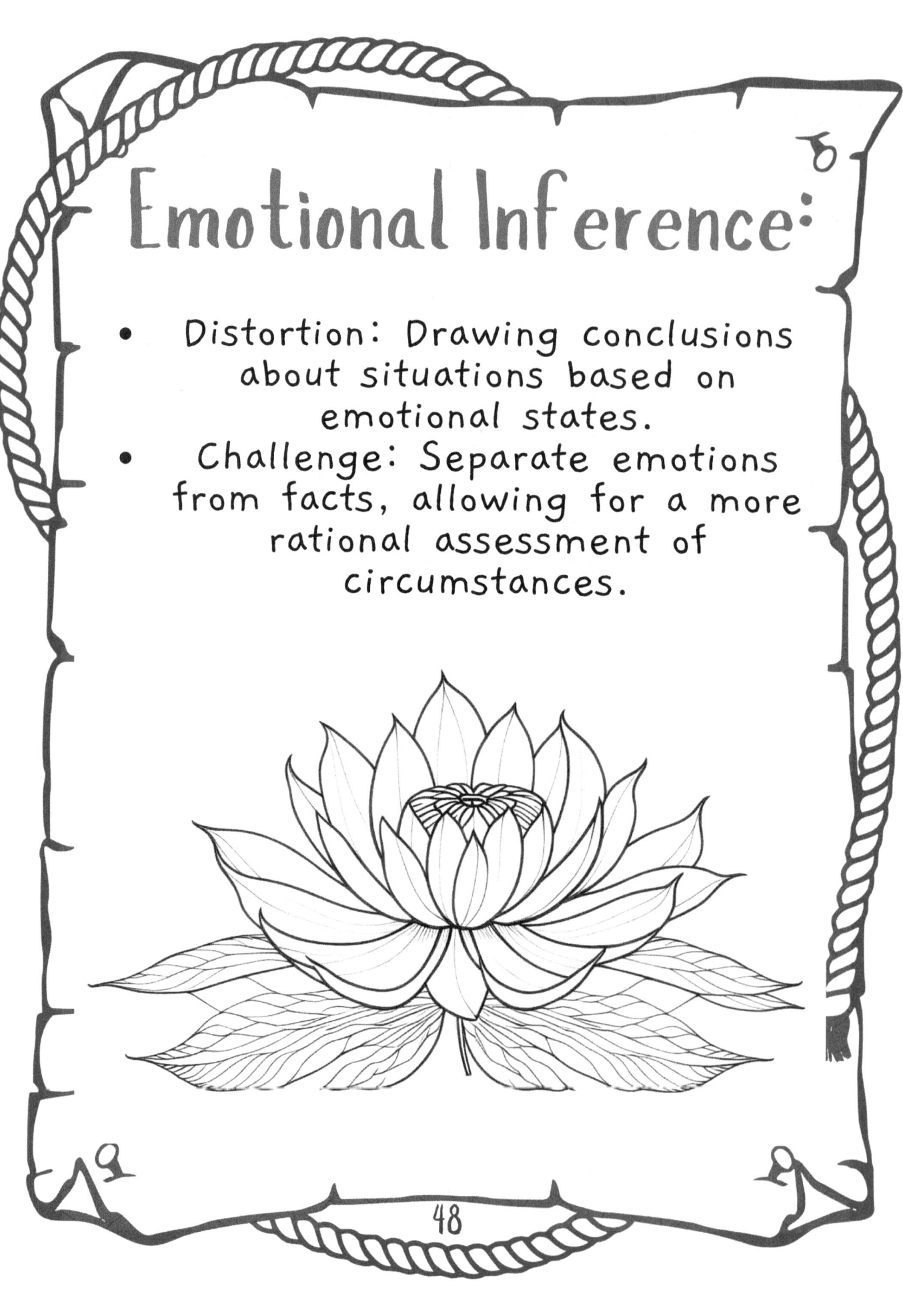

Comparing Inner Emotions to External Expectations:

- Distortion: Believing your emotions should always align with societal expectations.
- Challenge: Acknowledge and validate your emotions, recognizing that they are valid expressions of your experience.

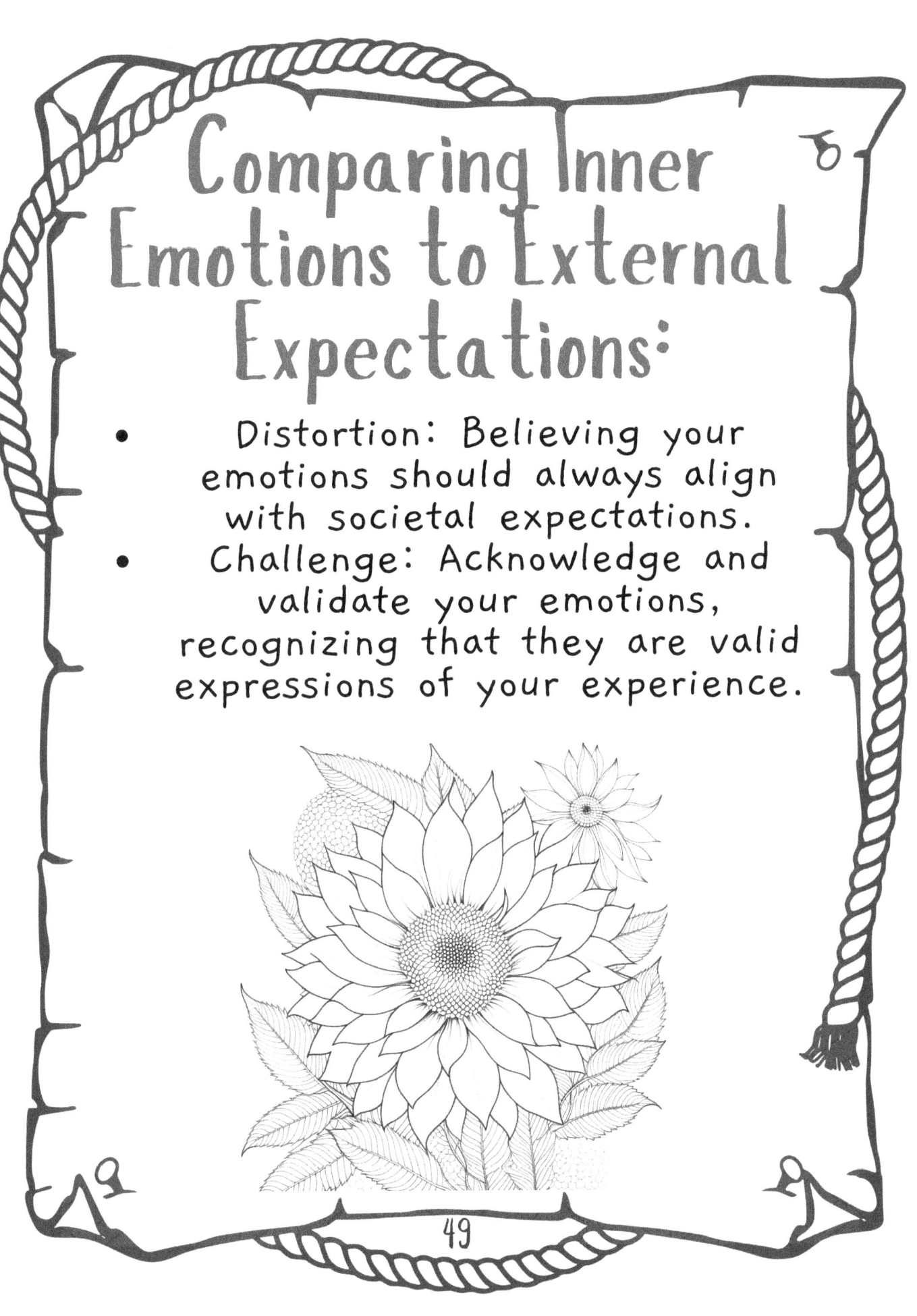

Selective Predicting:

- Distortion: Predicting outcomes based only on negative expectations.
- Challenge: Consider alternative, more balanced predictions, taking into account positive possibilities..

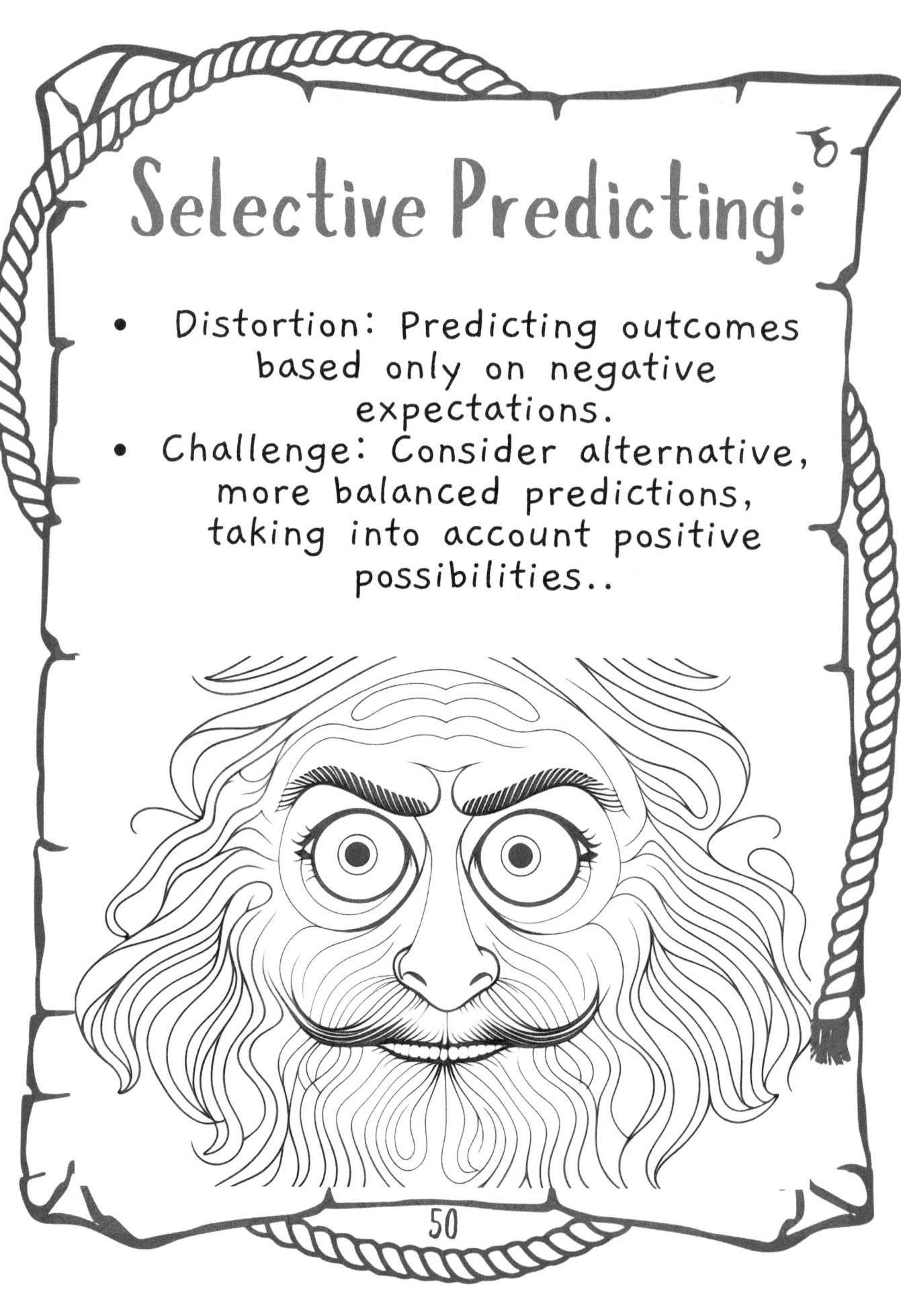

Perseveration:

- Distortion: Getting stuck on one thought or idea and unable to shift focus.
- Challenge: Practice mindfulness to redirect your attention and break the cycle of perseveration.

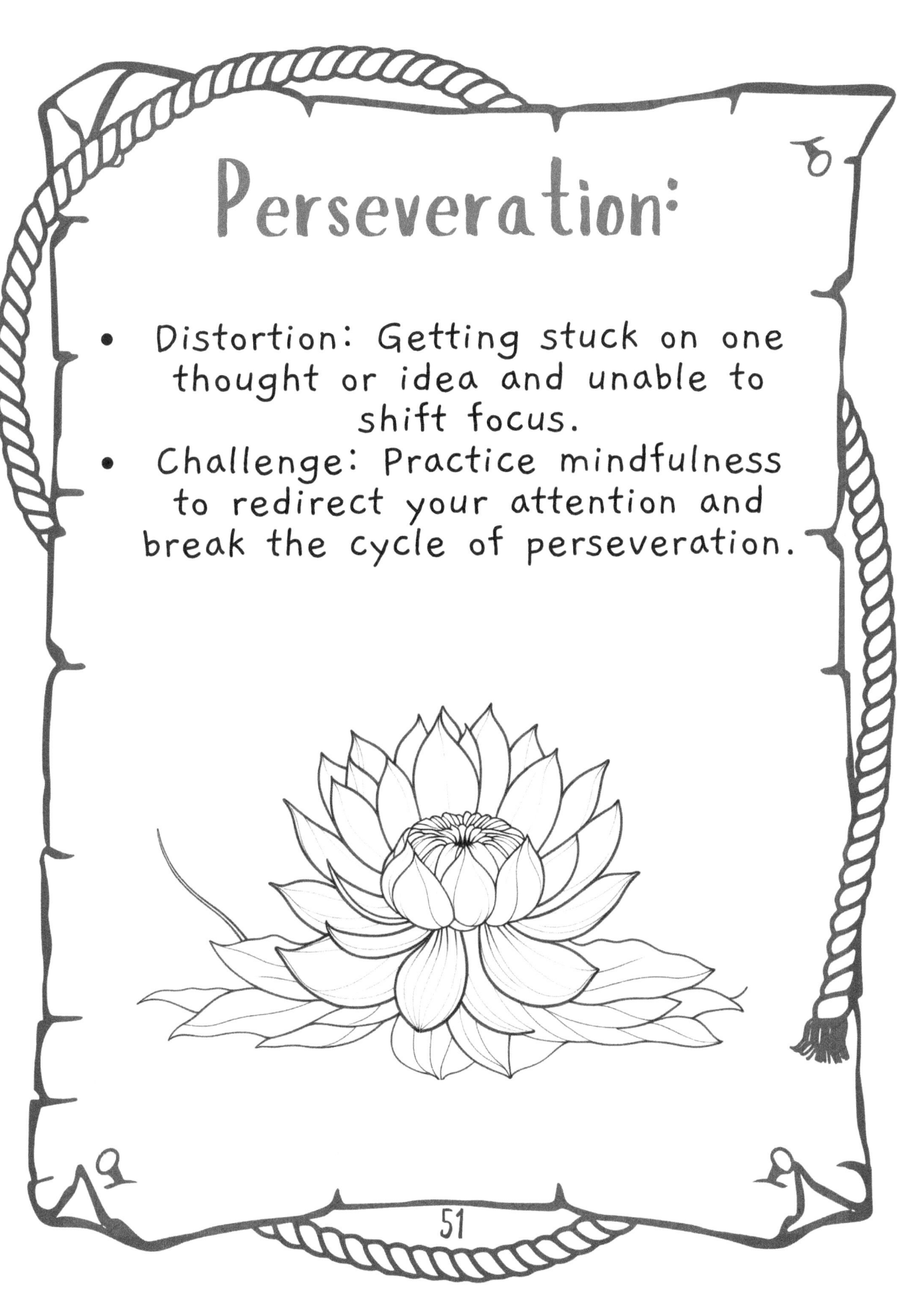

Assuming Others' Motivations:

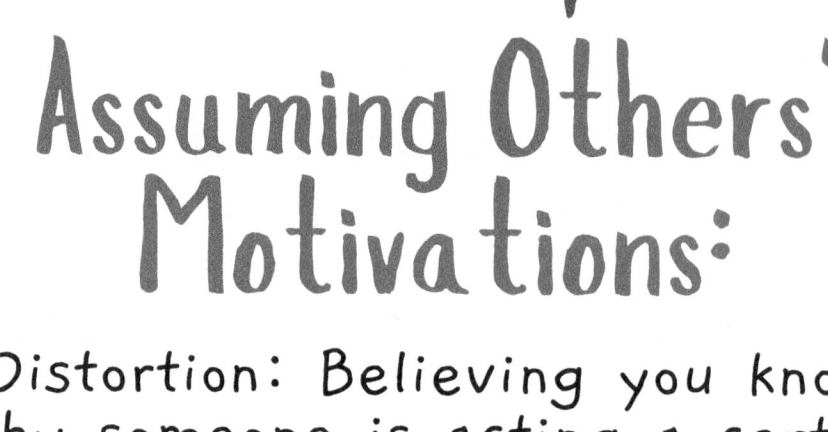

- Distortion: Believing you know why someone is acting a certain way without concrete evidence.
- Challenge: Communicate openly with others to understand their motivations rather than making assumptions.

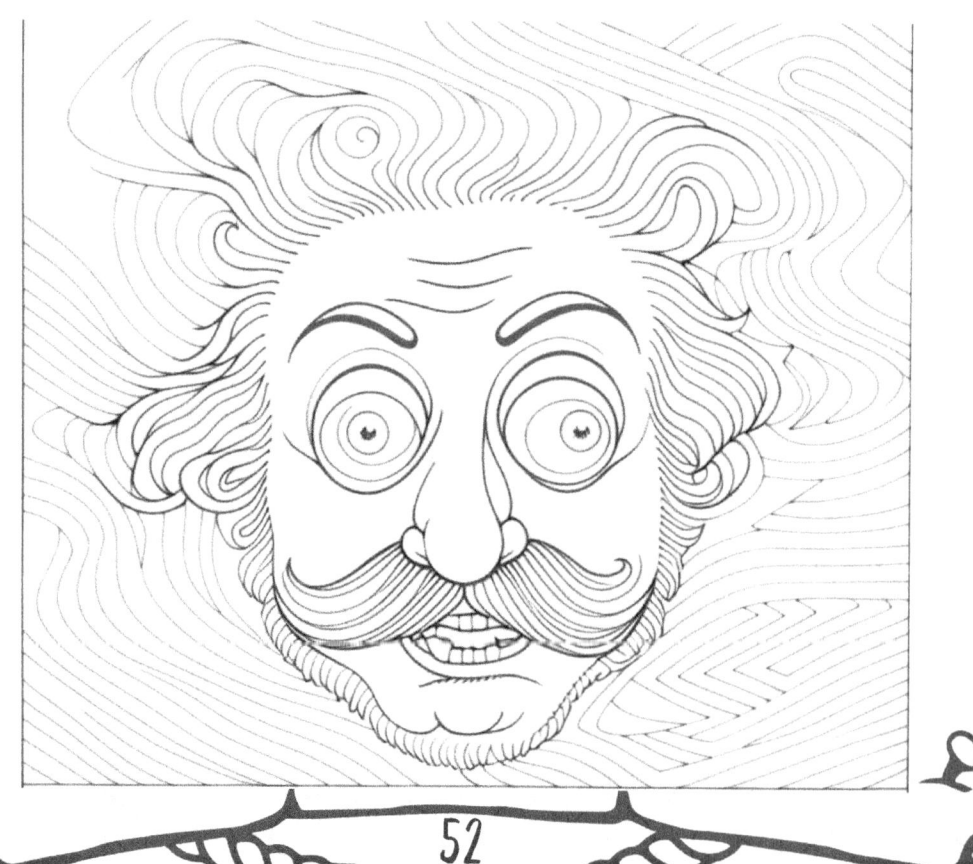

Personal Fable:

- Distortion: Feeling that your experiences are unique and others can't understand.
- Challenge: Recognize commonalities in human experiences, fostering connection and empathy.

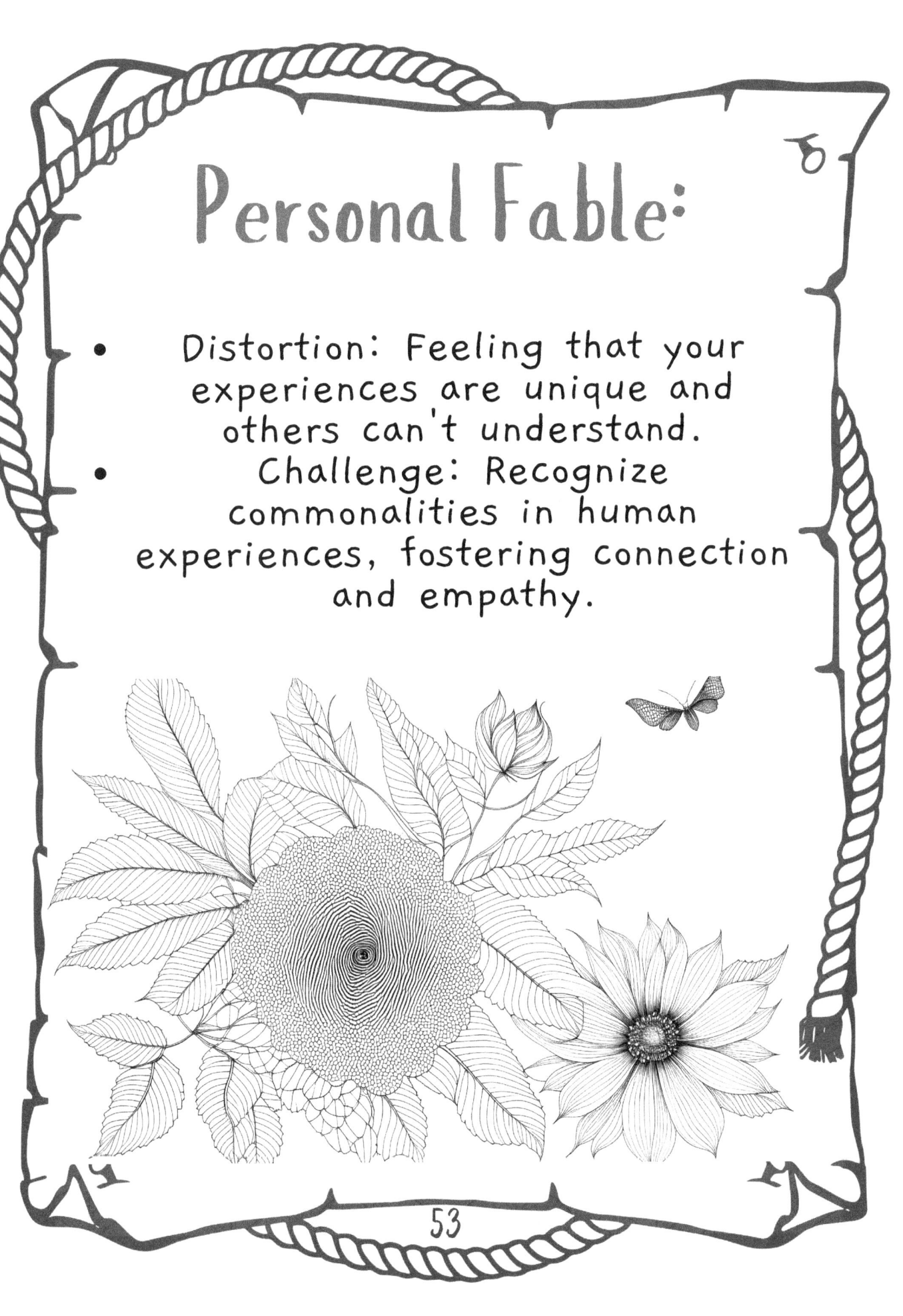

External Locus of Control:

- Distortion: Believing that external factors have complete control over your life.
- Challenge: Identify areas where you can exert influence and take proactive steps toward positive change.

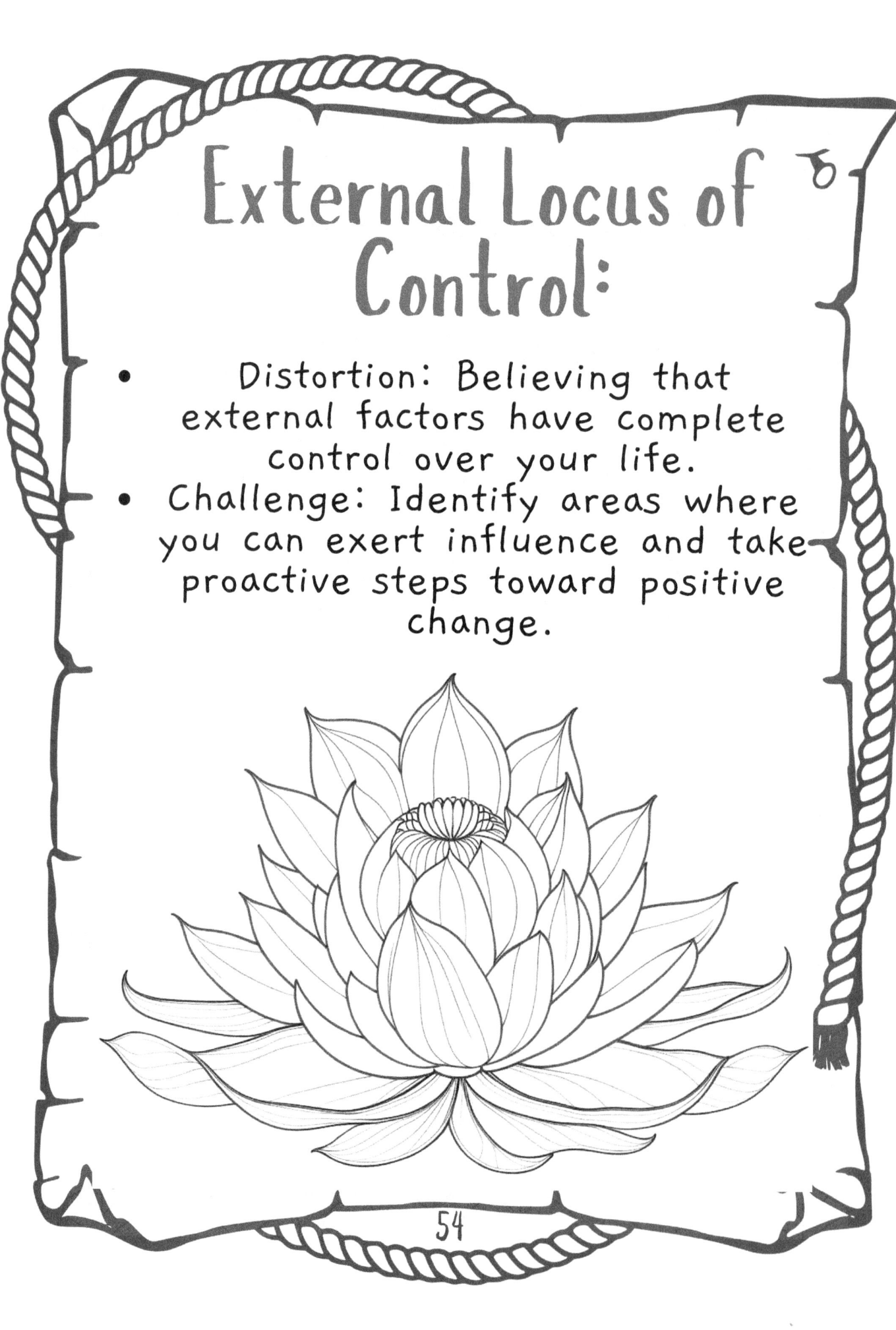

Inability to Distinguish Facts from Interpretations:

- Distortion: Blurring the line between facts and your interpretations of them.
- Challenge: Differentiate between objective facts and your subjective interpretations to foster clarity.

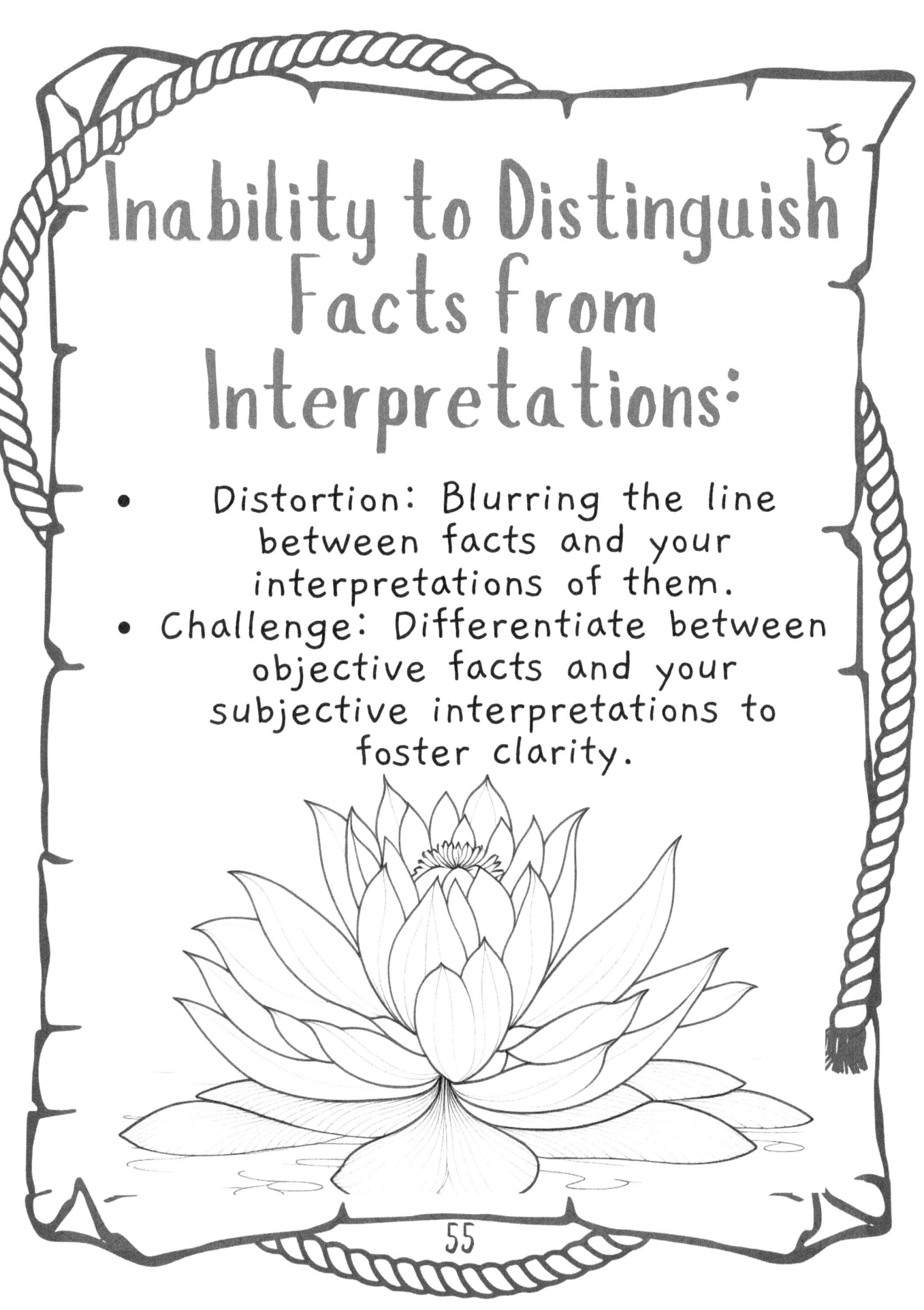

Chronic Self-Comparison:

- Distortion: Continuously measuring your achievements against others.
- Challenge: Set personal goals based on your values and celebrate your progress, regardless of others' achievements.

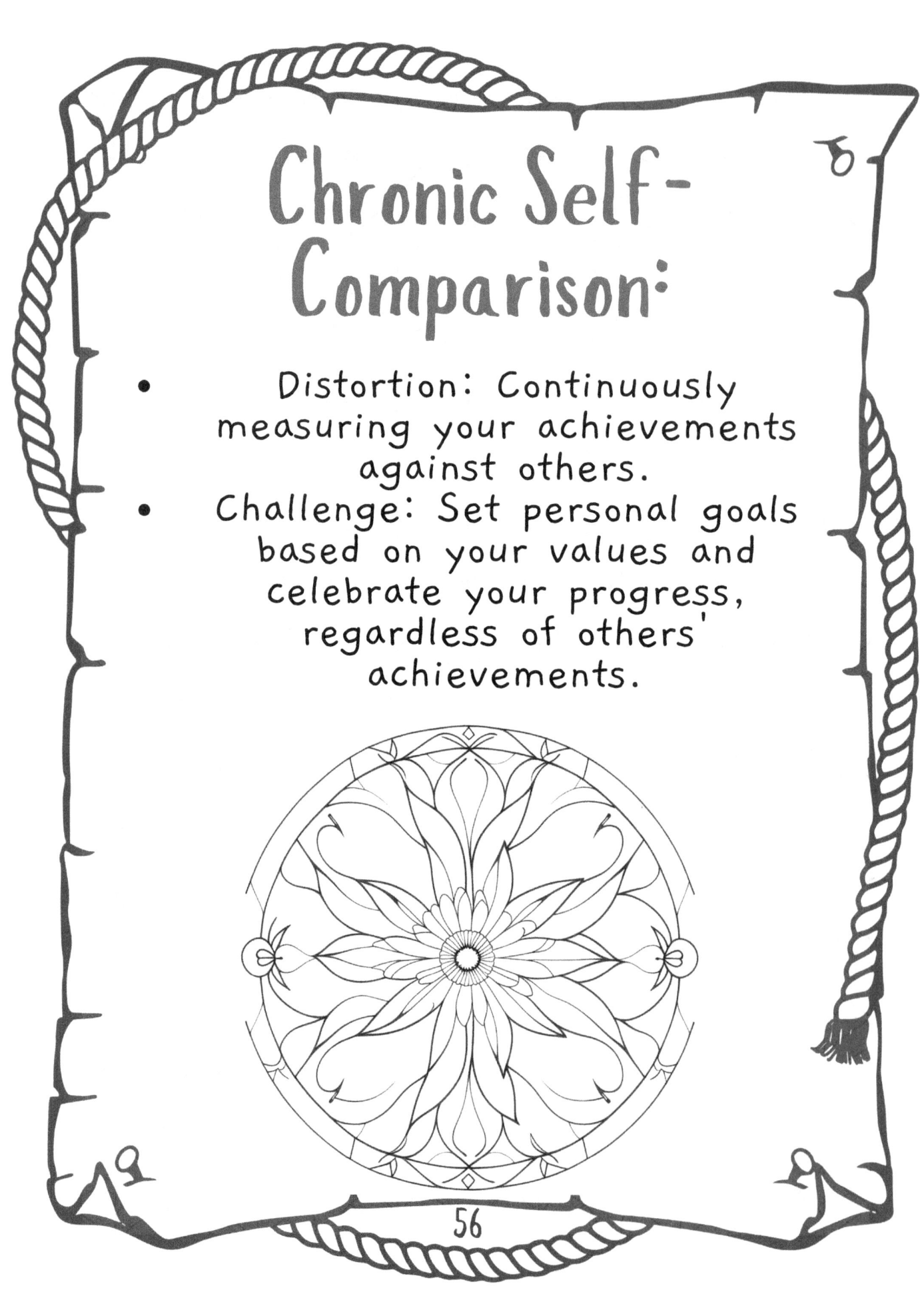

Cognitive Fusion:

- Distortion: Identifying too closely with your thoughts, as if they define you.
- Challenge: Practice observing your thoughts without necessarily identifying with them, promoting a healthier relationship with your mental processes.

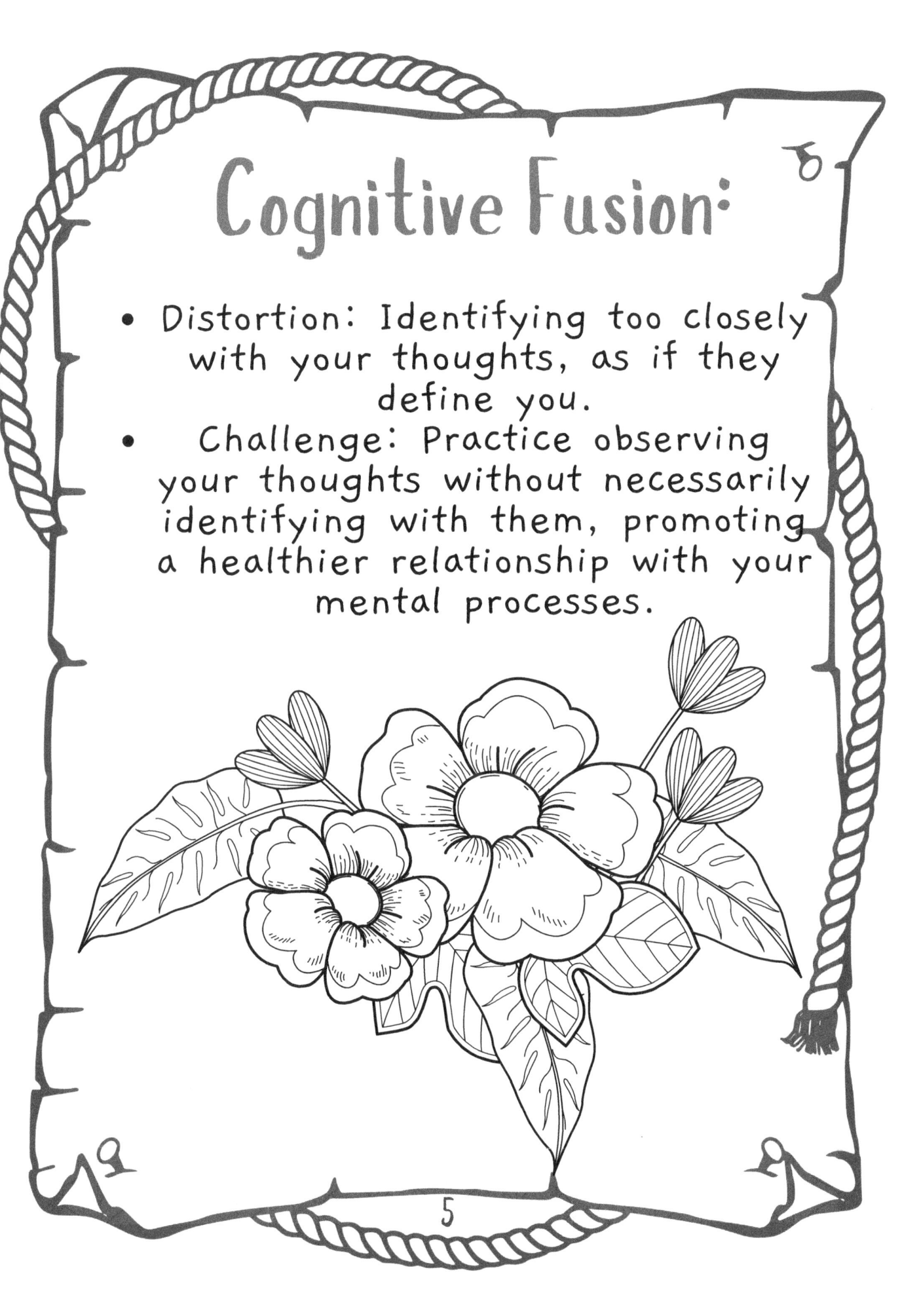

Overemphasis on Future Happiness:

- Distortion: Believing happiness is only attainable in the future, not in the present.
- Challenge: Cultivate gratitude for the positive aspects of your current circumstances, fostering a more content mindset.

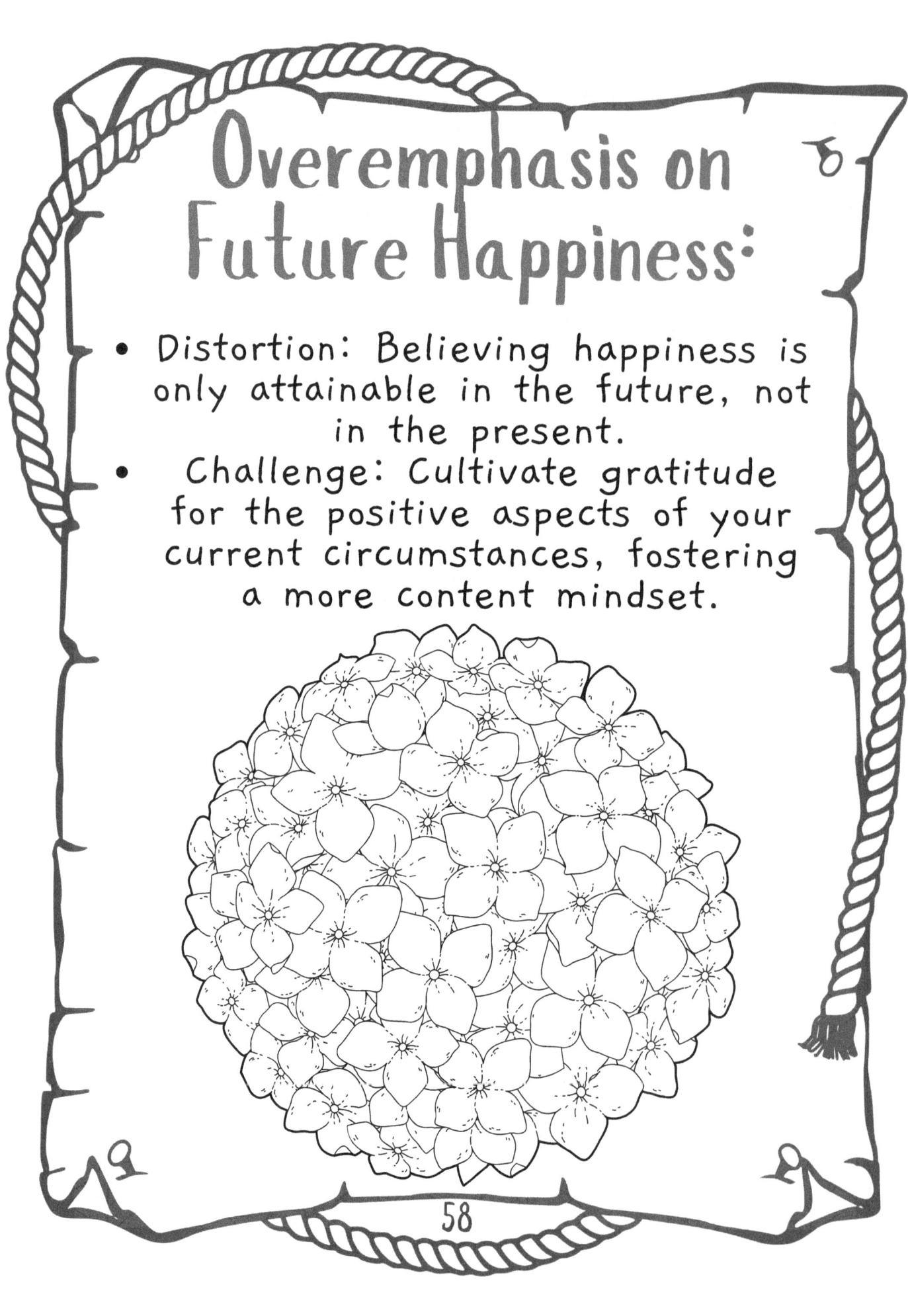

Expecting Others to Mind-Read:

- Distortion: Assuming others should know what you need without clear communication.
- Challenge: Express your thoughts and needs openly, facilitating better understanding in your relationships.

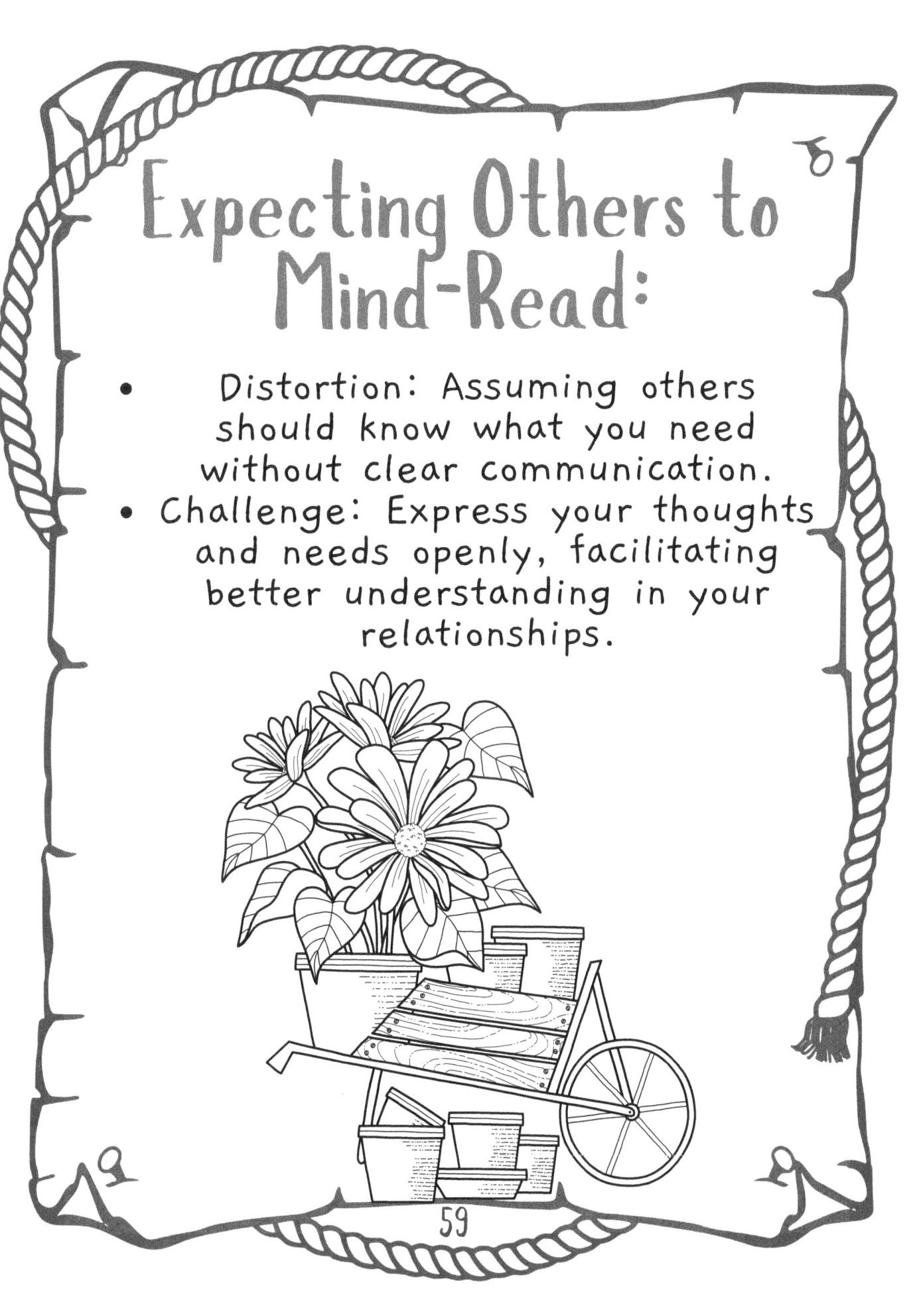

Future Tripping:

- Distortion: Excessively worrying about future events that may never occur.
- Challenge: Focus on the present moment and address challenges as they arise, rather than getting lost in hypothetical scenarios.

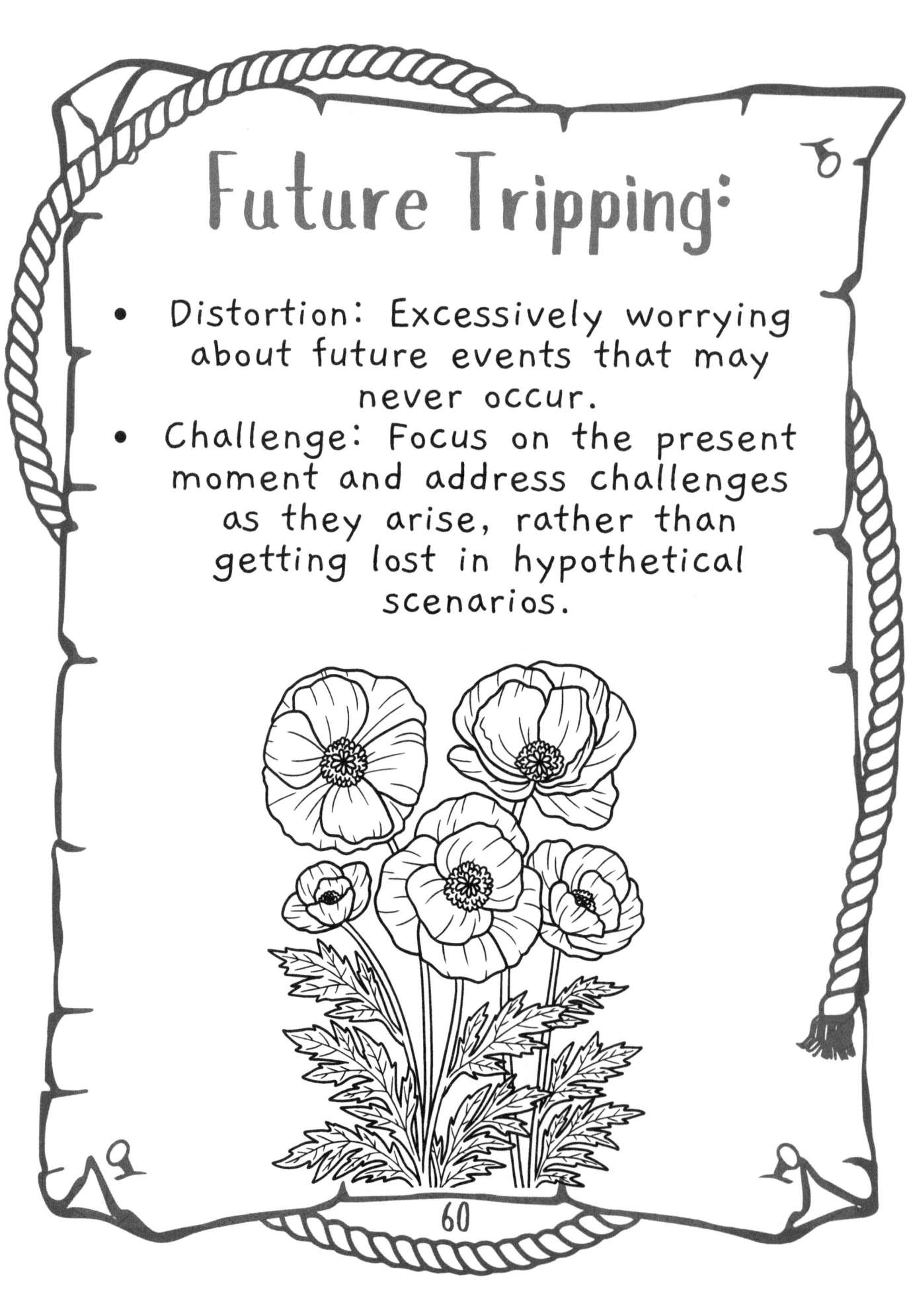

Selective Gratitude:

- Distortion: Acknowledging only negative aspects of a situation while ignoring positive elements.
- Challenge: Practice gratitude by consciously noting and appreciating positive aspects, no matter how small.

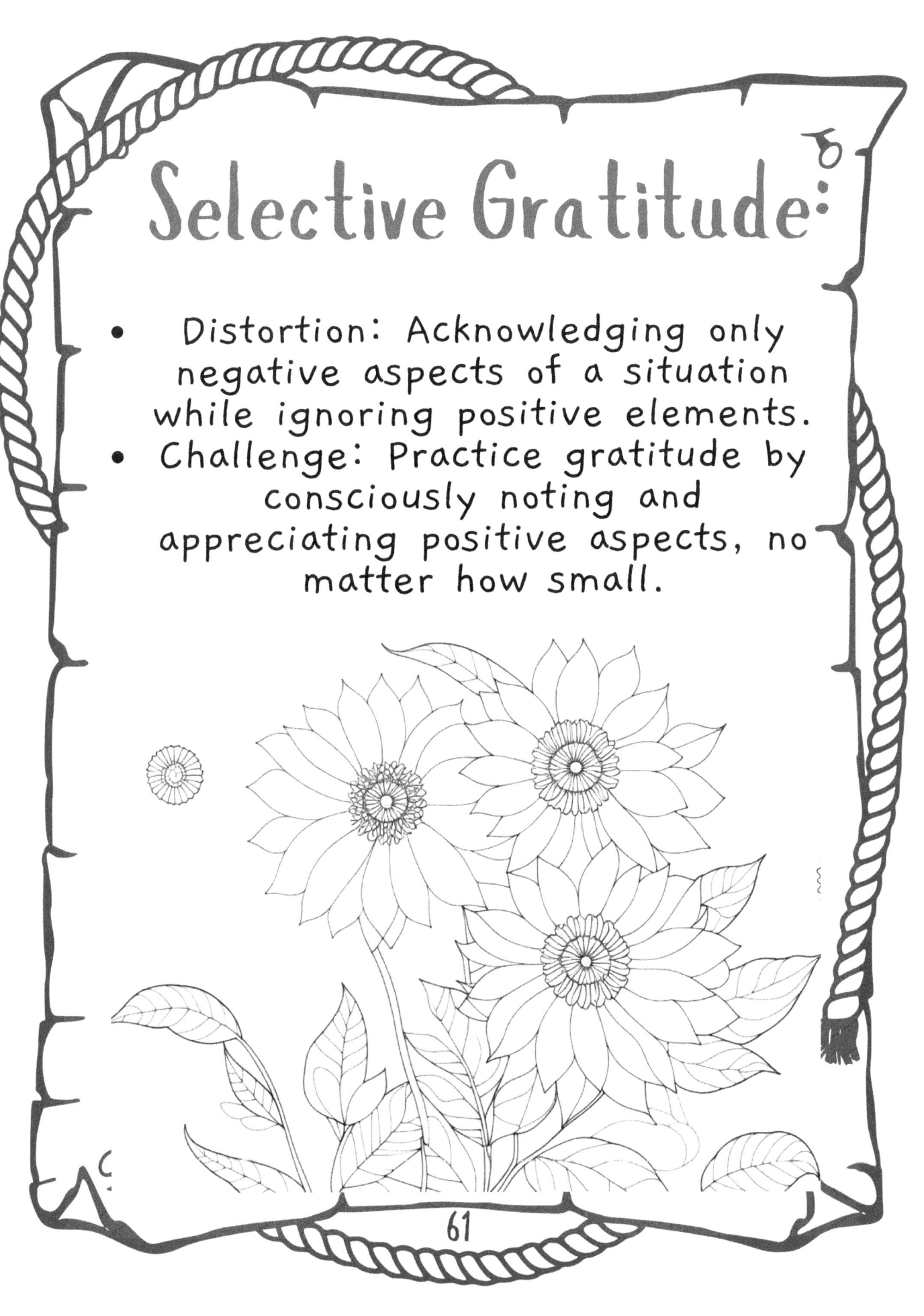

Projection:

- Distortion: Attributing your own feelings or characteristics to others.
- Challenge: Be mindful of projecting your emotions onto others; consider alternative perspectives.

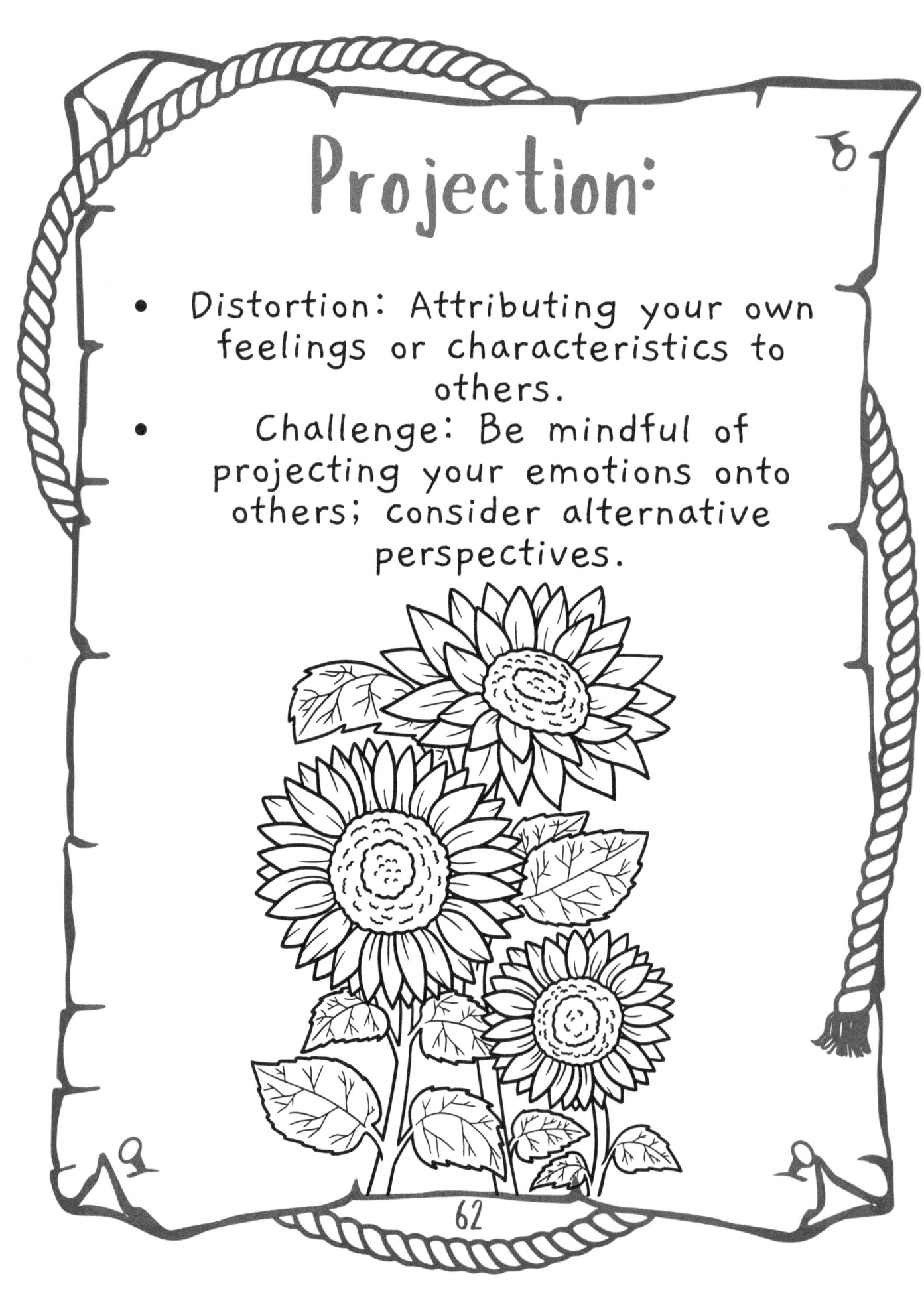

Expecting Others to Mind-Read:

- Distortion: Assuming others should know what you need without clear communication.
- Challenge: Express your thoughts and needs openly, facilitating better understanding in your relationships.

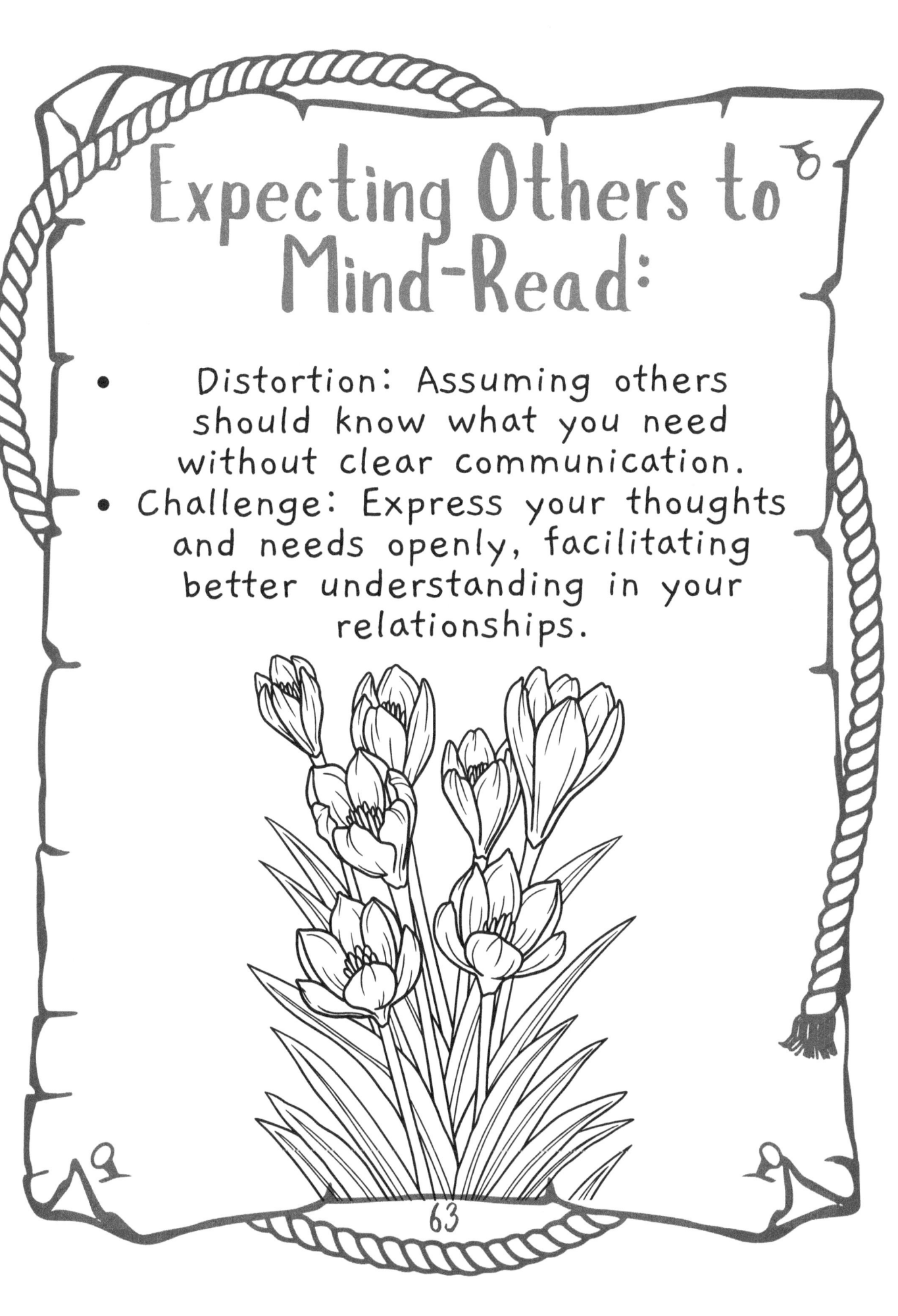

Dehumanization:

- Distortion: Viewing yourself or others as less than human, often in times of conflict.
- Challenge: Foster empathy by recognizing the shared humanity and complexities of individuals.

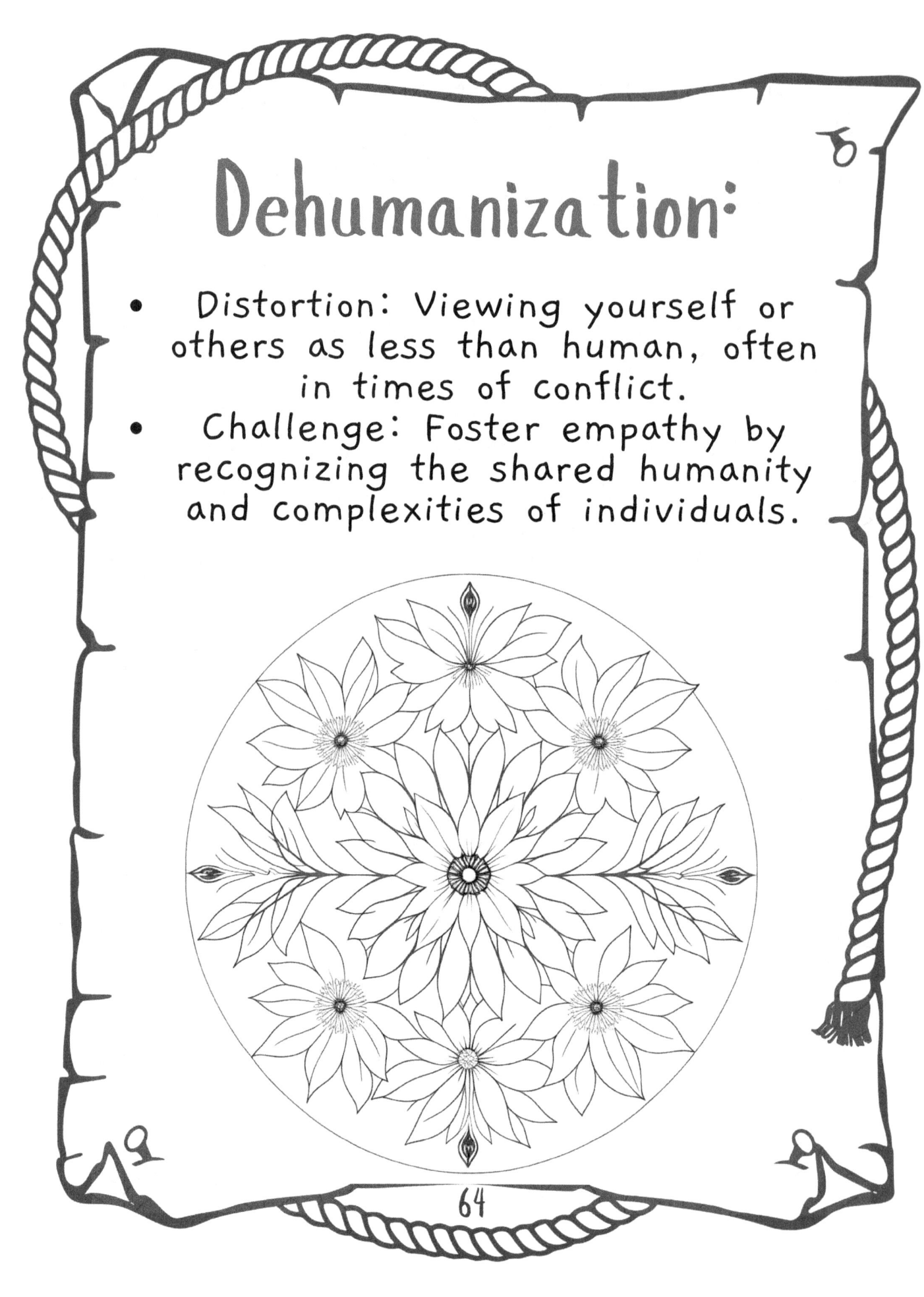

Escapism:

- Distortion: Avoiding reality by engaging in activities that provide temporary relief.
- Challenge: Confront challenges directly and develop healthier coping mechanisms to address stressors.

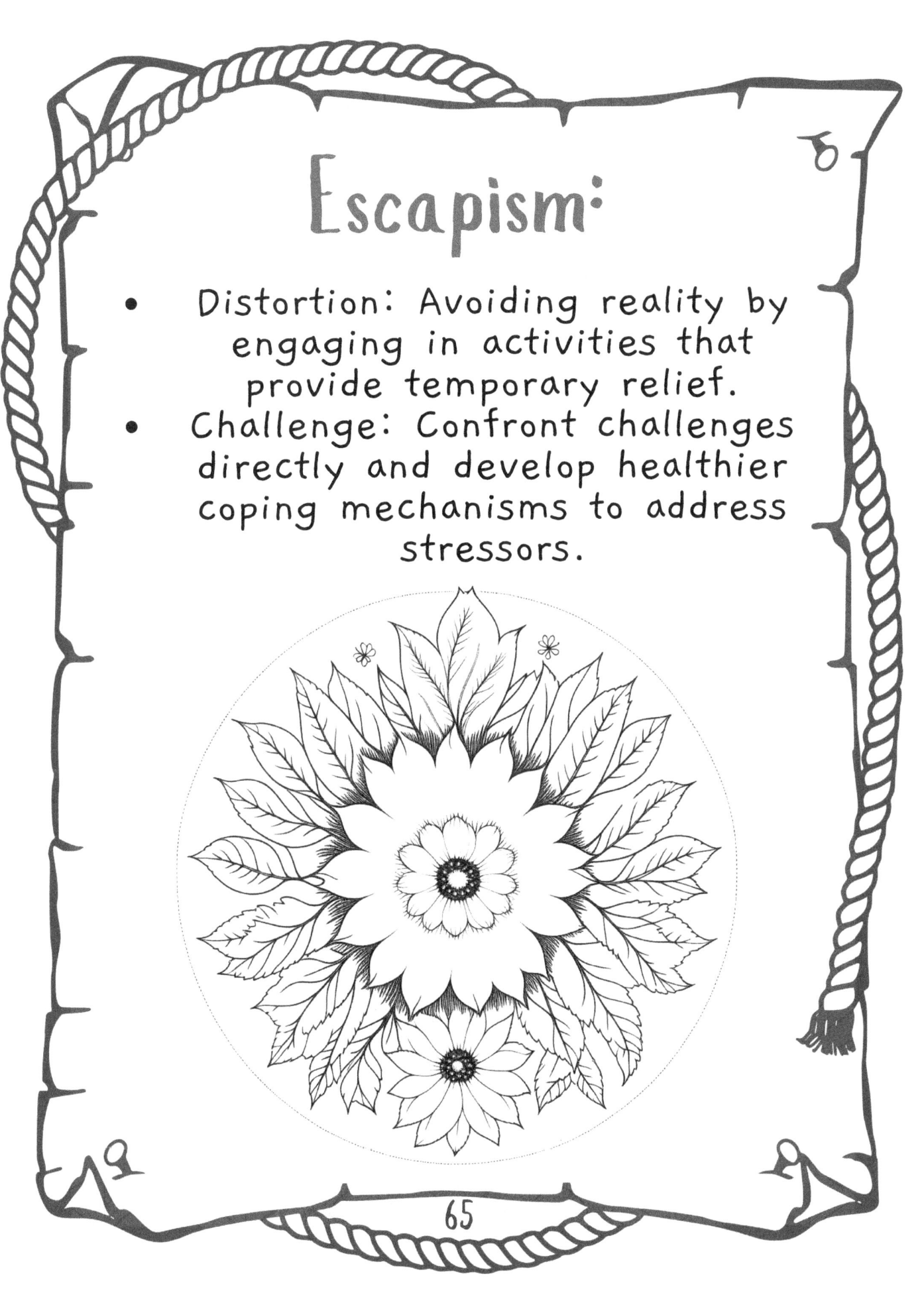

Self-Critical Perfectionism:

- Distortion: Setting unrealistic standards for yourself and harshly criticizing perceived failures.
- Challenge: Embrace the concept of progress over perfection and celebrate your efforts, not just the outcomes.

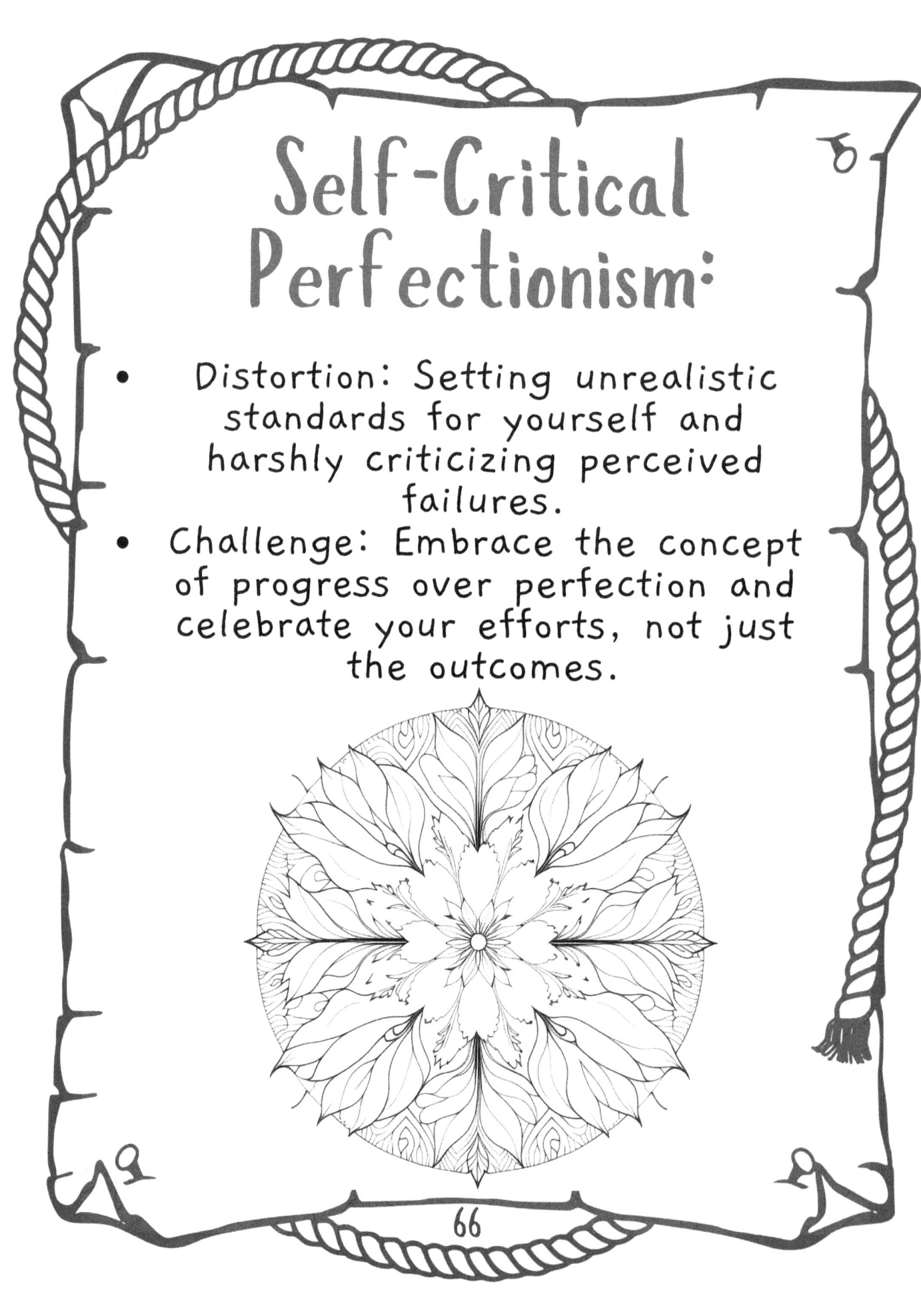

Comparing Inner Reality to External Image:

- Distortion: Assuming others' external appearances accurately represent their inner reality.
- Challenge: Recognize that everyone faces internal struggles, regardless of outward appearances.

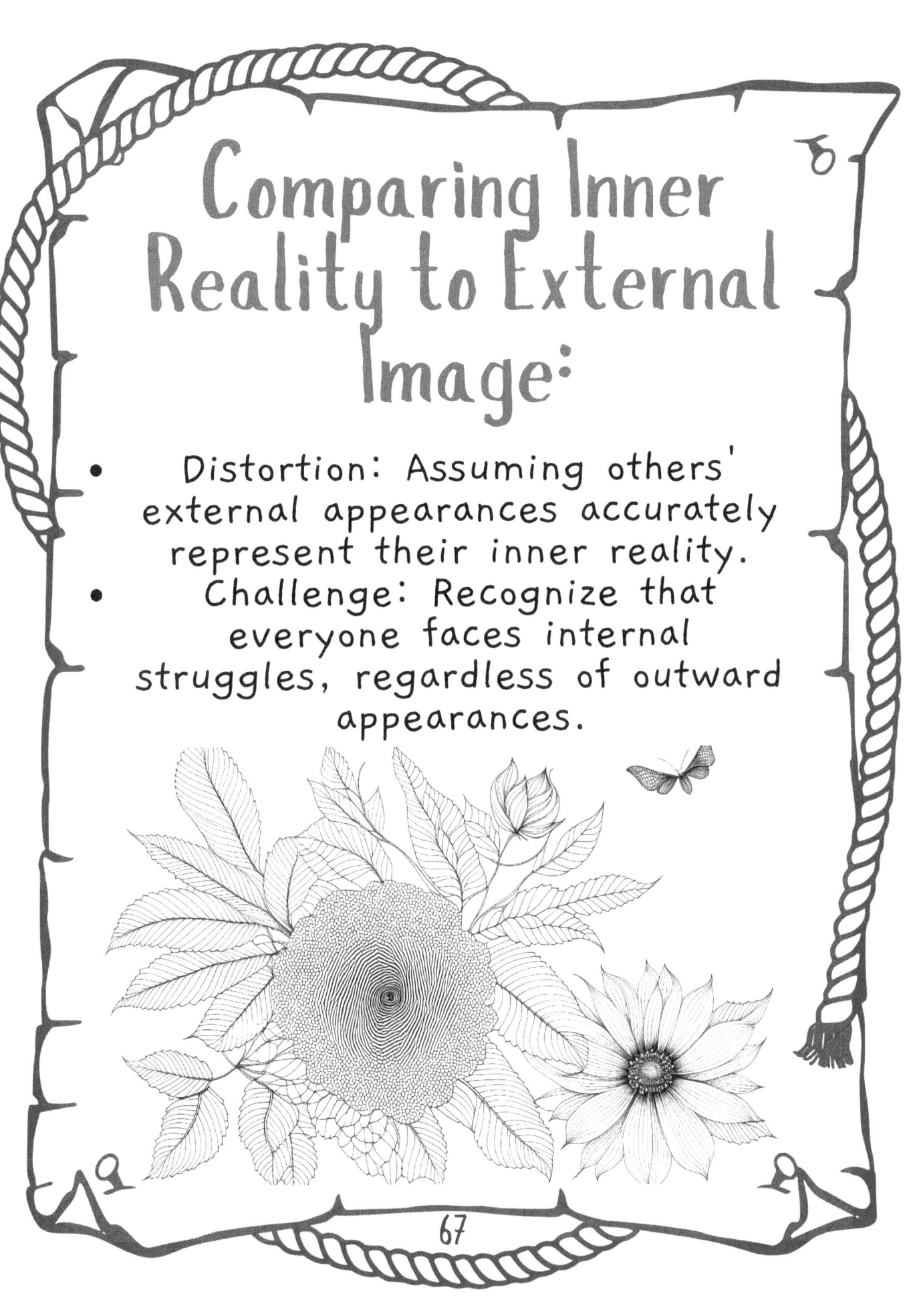

Present Moment Disregard:

- Distortion: Ignoring the importance of the present moment in pursuit of future goals.
- Challenge: Balance goal-setting with mindfulness, appreciating the significance of the current journey.

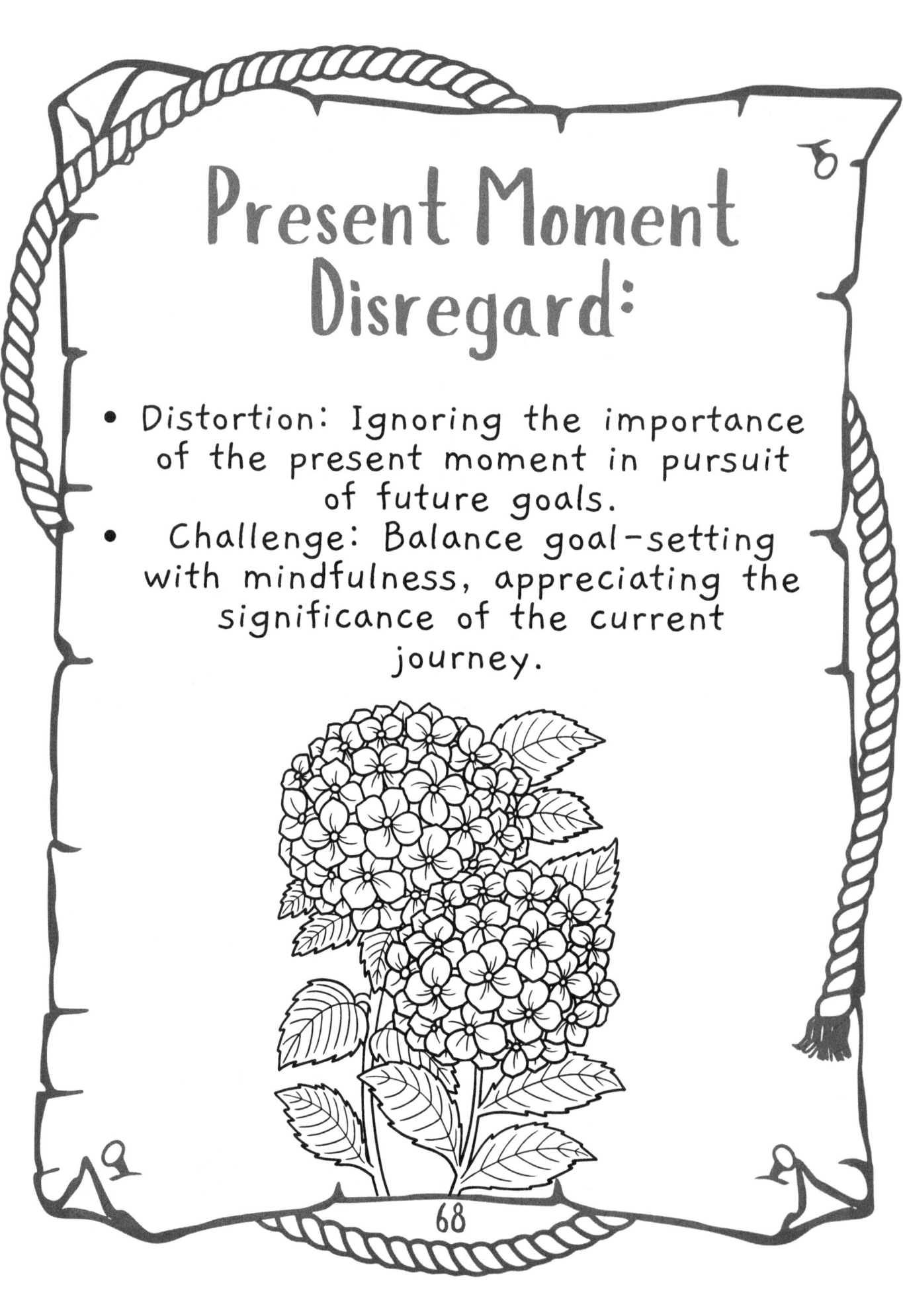

Overemphasis on Self-Reliance:

- Distortion: Believing you should handle everything on your own without seeking support.
- Challenge: Recognize the strength in seeking help and collaboration; it's a sign of resilience, not weakness.

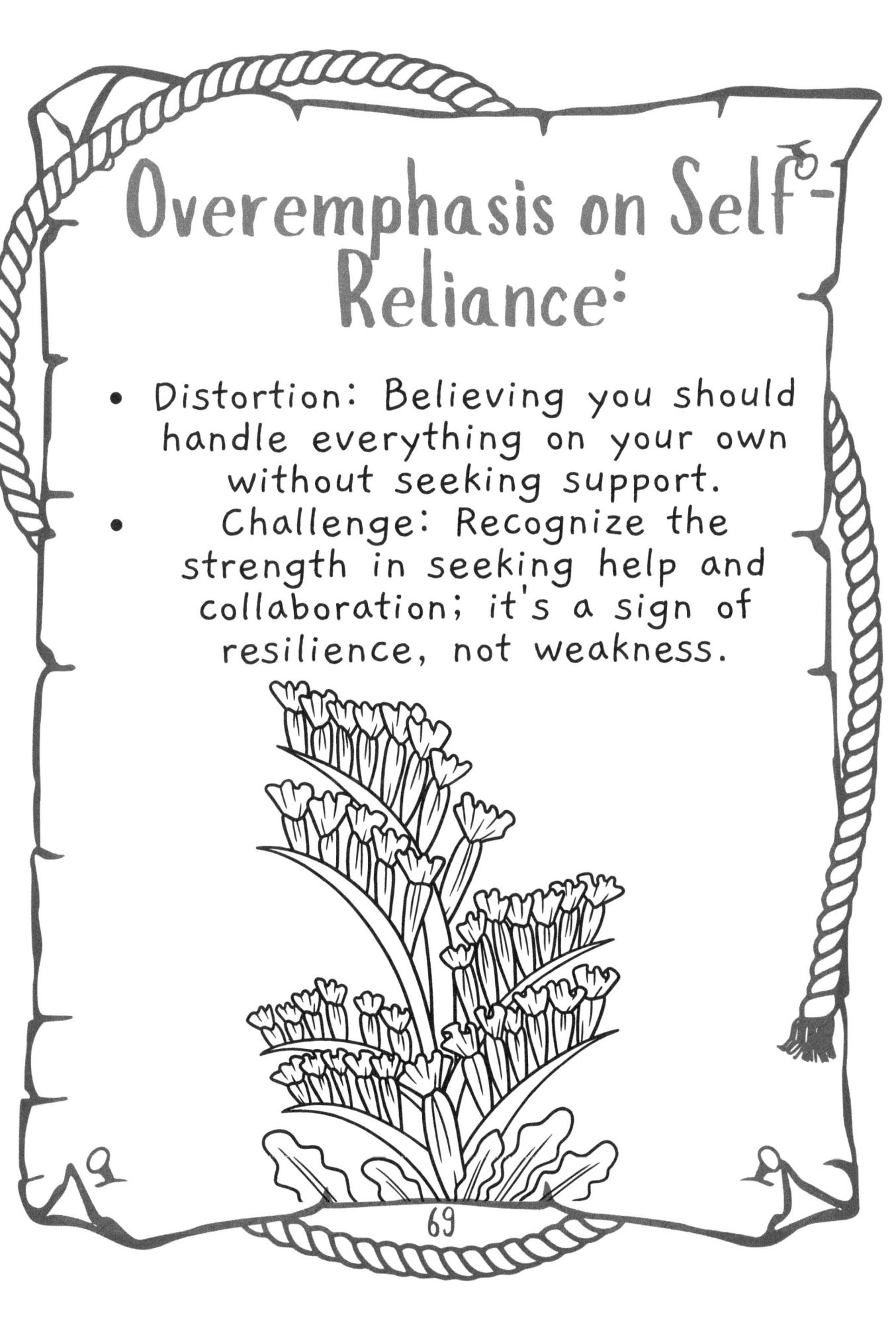

Overgeneralizing from Past Mistakes:

- Distortion: Assuming that because you made a mistake in the past, you'll inevitably repeat it.
- Challenge: Acknowledge the lessons learned from past experiences and use them as opportunities for growth.

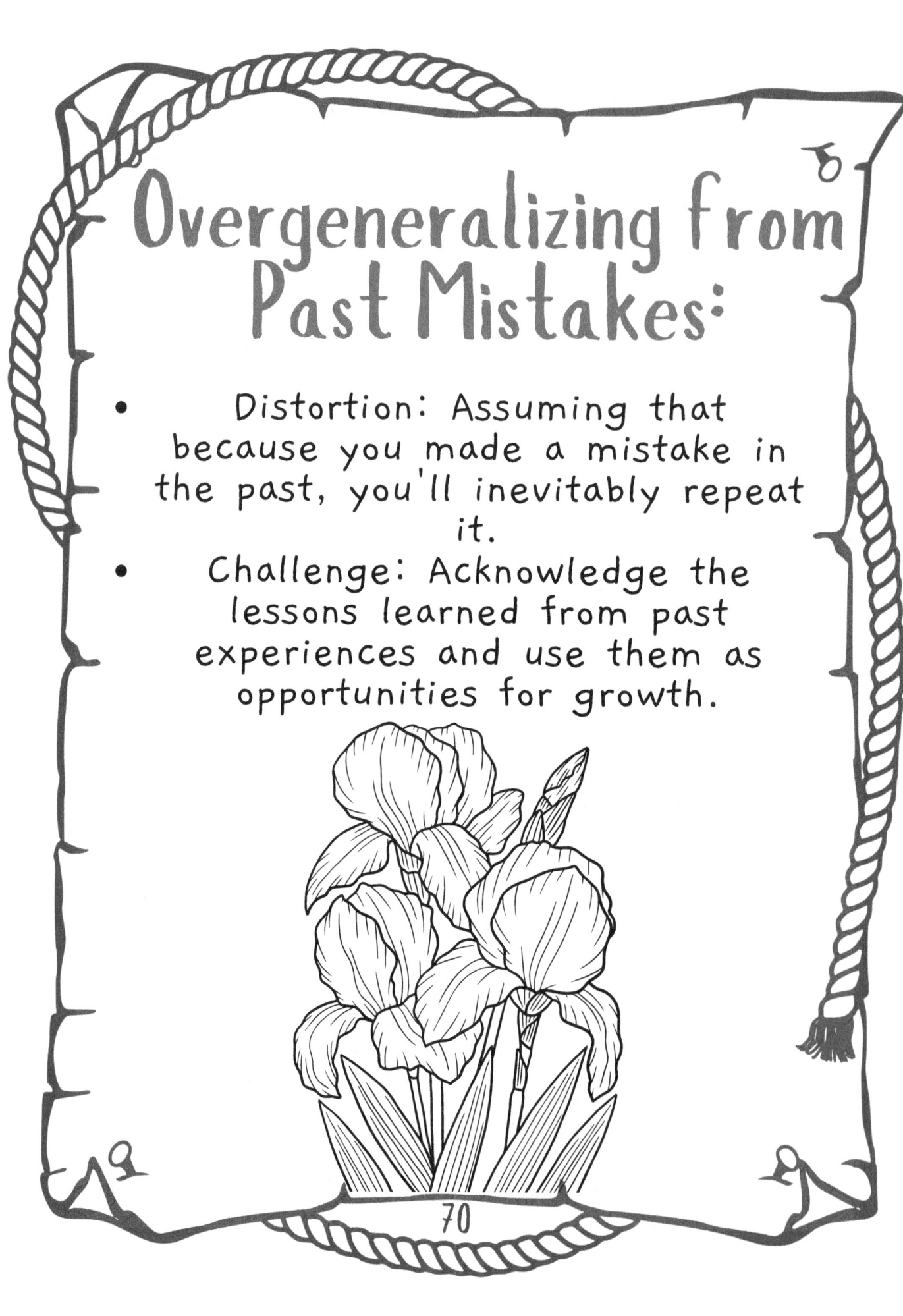

By recognizing these cognitive distortions and actively challenging them, you can develop a more balanced and realistic perspective, leading to improved mental well-being.

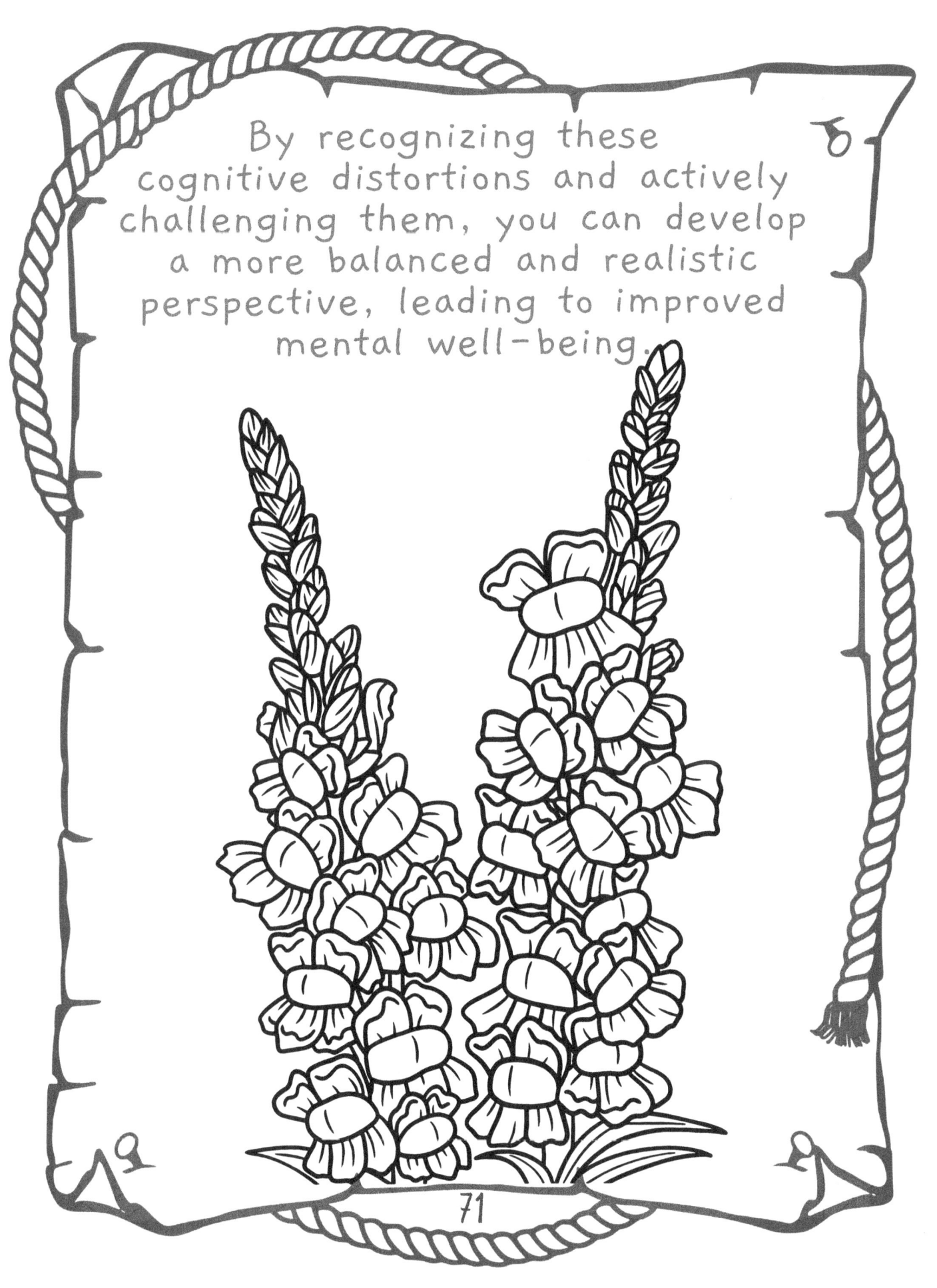

Remember, challenging cognitive distortions is an ongoing process that involves self-awareness and practice. Developing a habit of questioning negative thoughts and replacing them with more balanced perspectives can lead to significant improvements in mental well-being. If you find these distortions persisting or impacting your daily life, seeking professional guidance is a proactive step toward positive change.

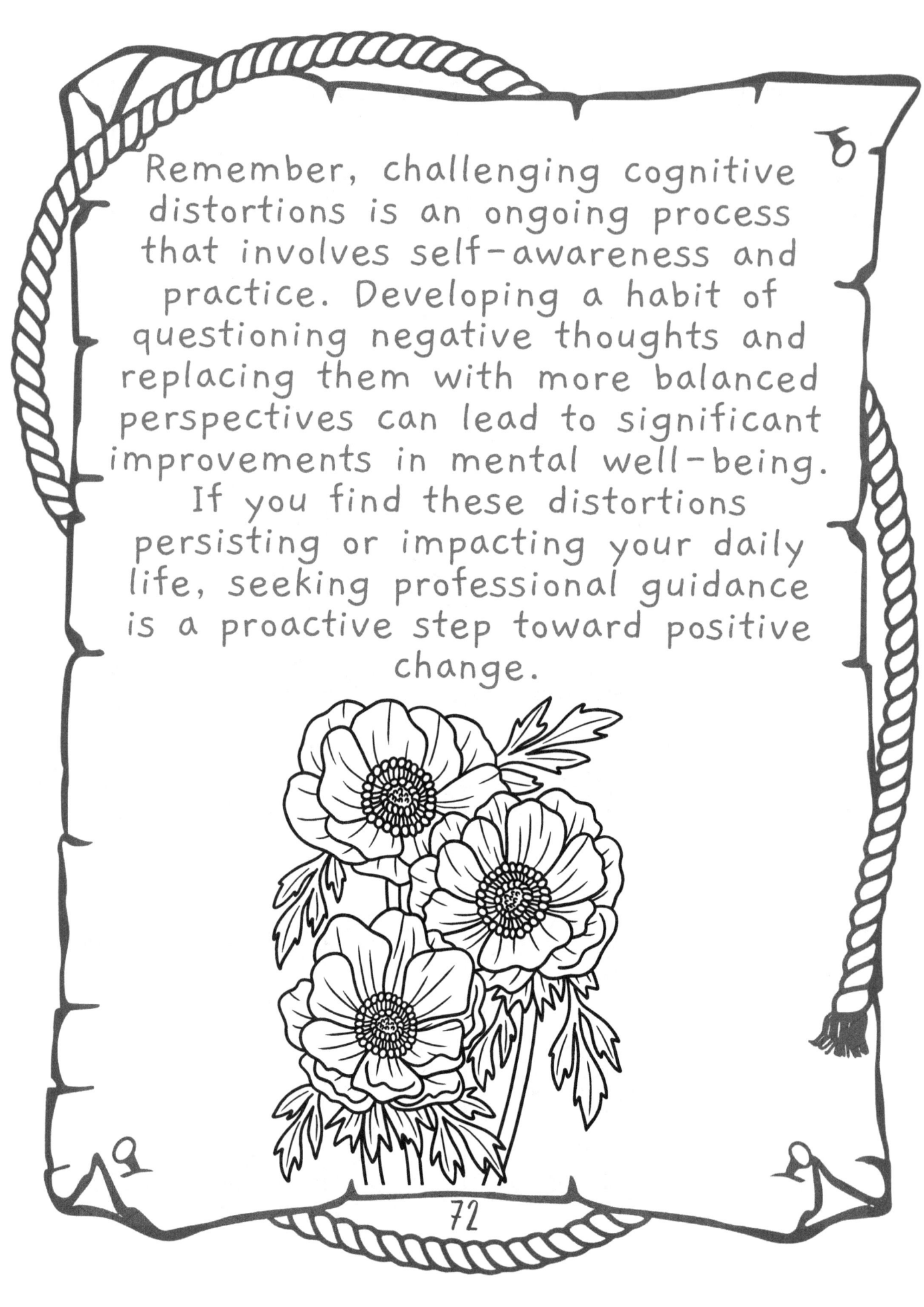

By understanding and challenging these cognitive distortions, you empower yourself to foster a more positive and realistic mindset. It's essential to cultivate self-compassion and patience during this process, as change takes time and consistent effort. If you find it challenging to navigate these distortions on your own, seeking guidance from a mental health professional can provide valuable support and strategies tailored to your specific needs.

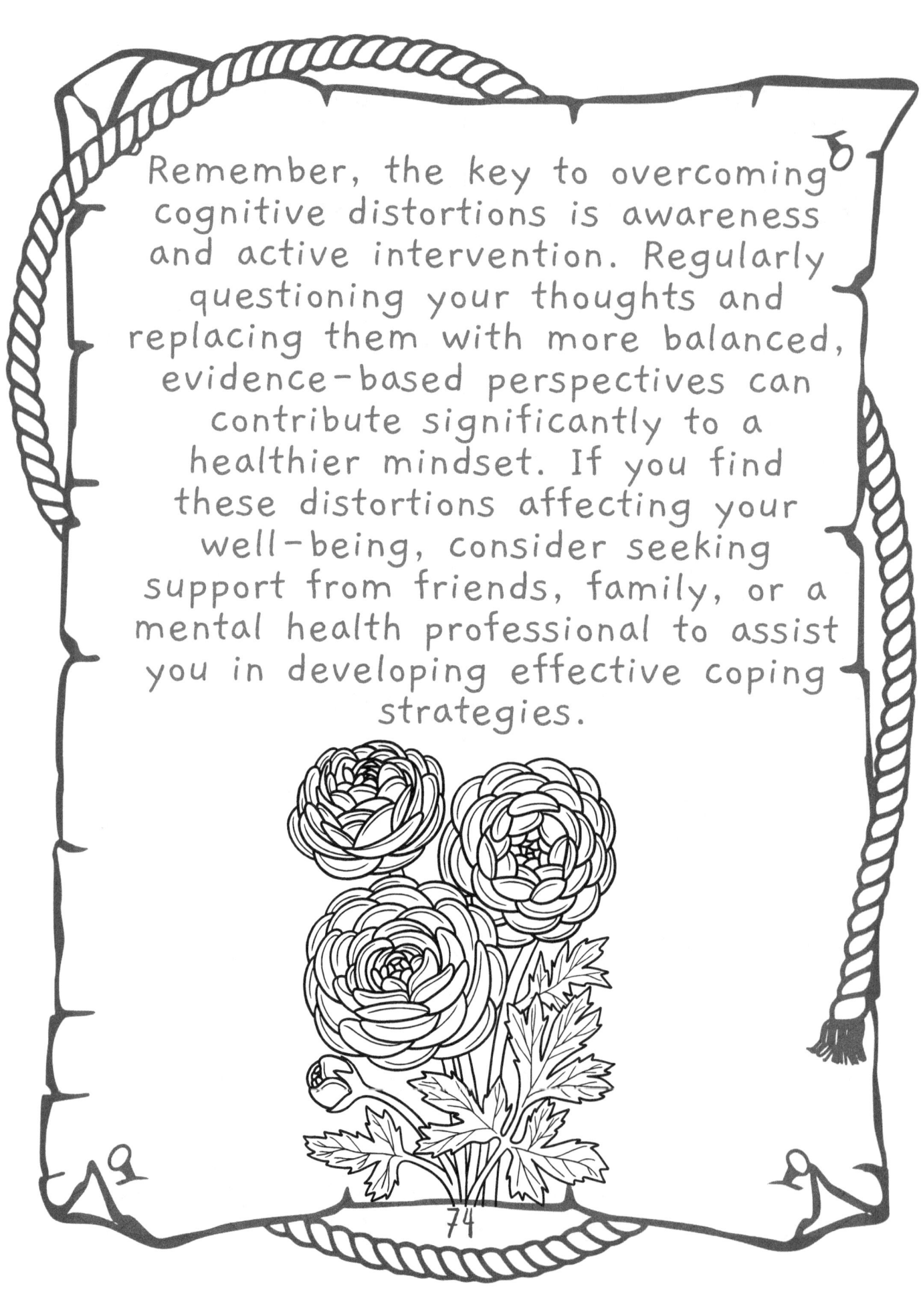

Remember, the key to overcoming cognitive distortions is awareness and active intervention. Regularly questioning your thoughts and replacing them with more balanced, evidence-based perspectives can contribute significantly to a healthier mindset. If you find these distortions affecting your well-being, consider seeking support from friends, family, or a mental health professional to assist you in developing effective coping strategies.

Remember, the journey to challenging cognitive distortions involves continuous self-reflection and a commitment to cultivating a more balanced perspective. If you find these distortions persisting or impacting your daily life, seeking professional guidance is a proactive step toward positive change.

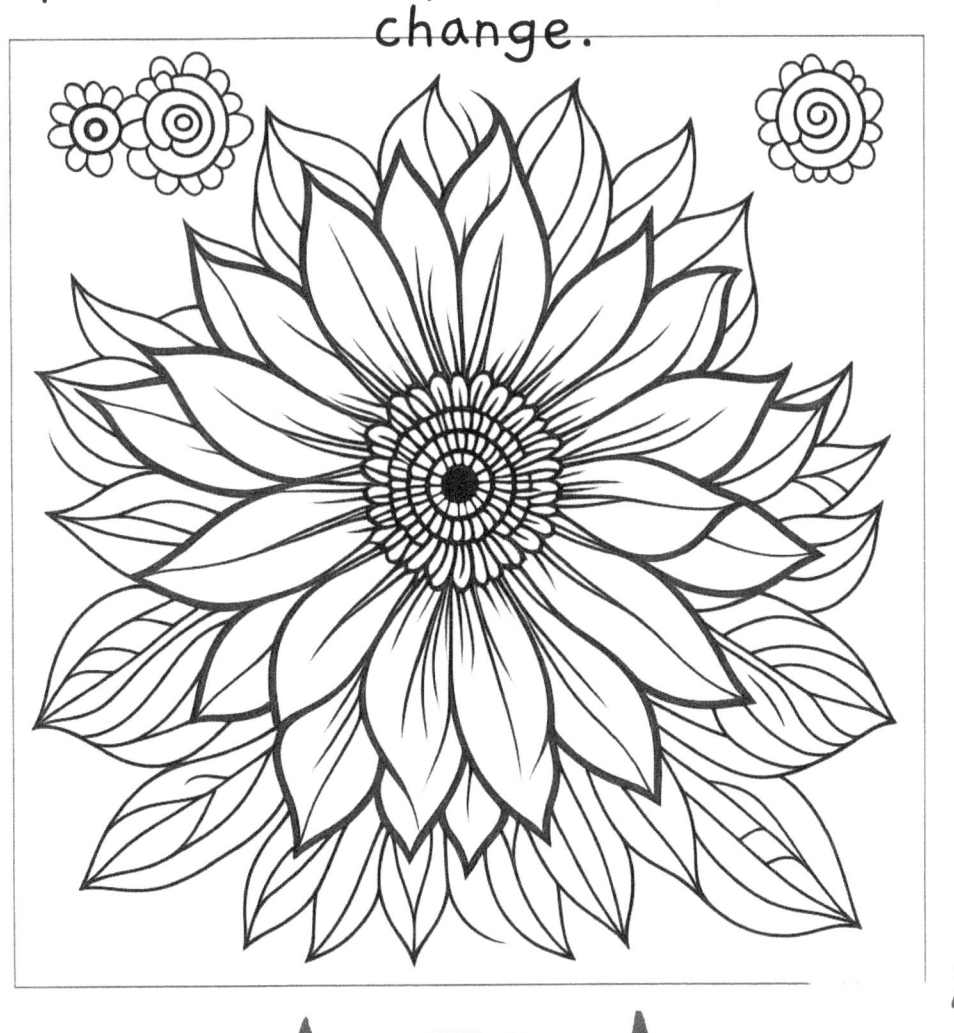

As you continue to explore and challenge these cognitive distortions, remember that self-compassion and patience are essential. Developing a habit of questioning negative thoughts and fostering a more balanced perspective can contribute significantly to improved mental well-being. If you find these distortions persisting or impacting your daily life, seeking professional guidance is a proactive step toward positive change.

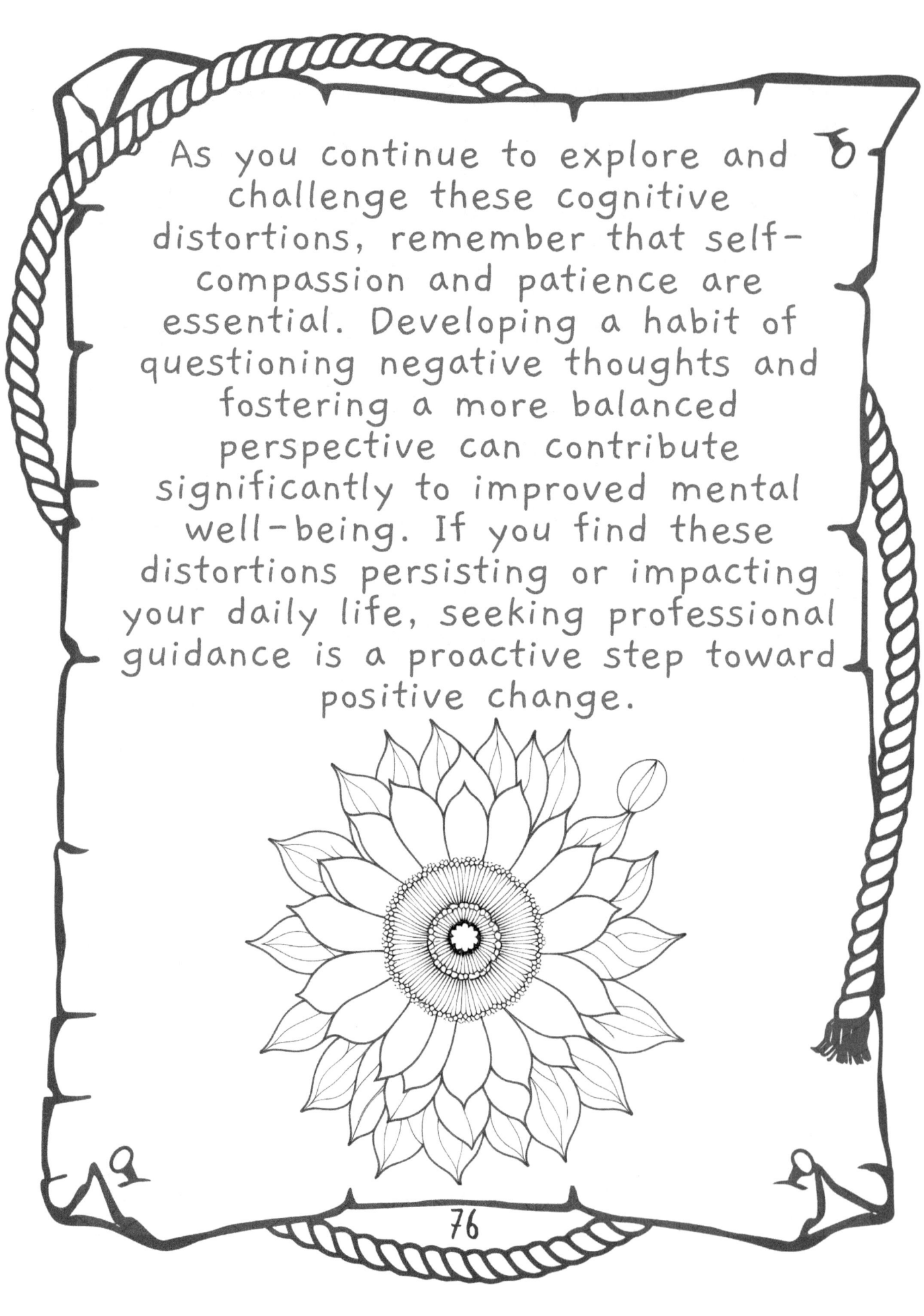

MANDALA
COLORING

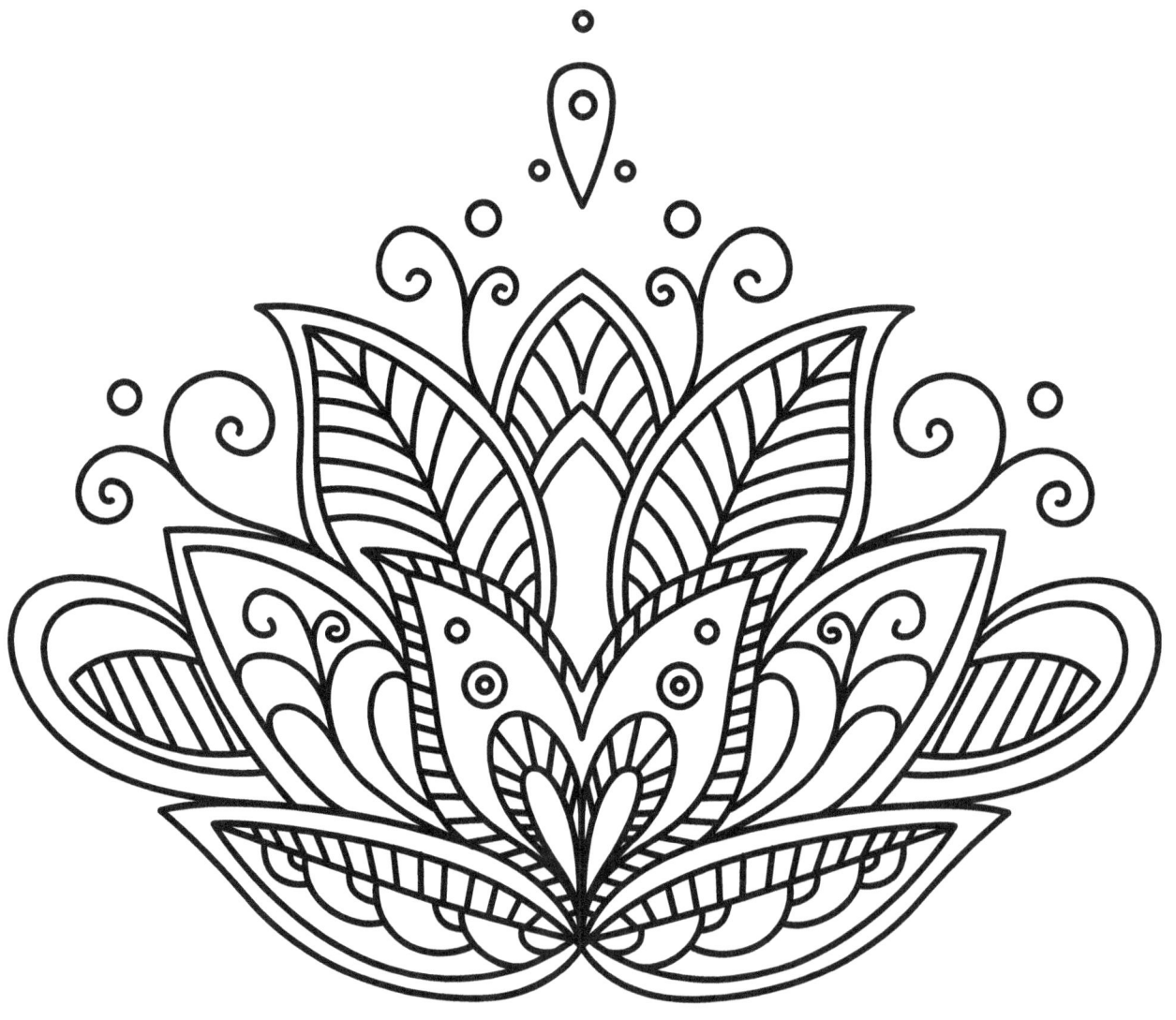

www.ingramcontent.com/pod-product-compliance
Lightning Source LLC
Chambersburg PA
CBHW082145290526
45794CB00008B/3172